LIVE AS IF...

"If a love had a voice and could tell us its story, it would be this one by Frye Gaillard. As Gaillard recounts the extraordinary life of his wife, Nancy, he honors her in revealing her heroism as a teacher, chronicling her resilience, and portraying the courage of her everyday choices and actions. In spirited and generous prose, Gaillard offers us a peek into a life so well-lived, a life so full of courage and generosity, that it changes us just by reading about her."

—Patti Callahan Henry, Author of *Becoming Mrs. Lewis*, winner of the Harper Lee Award

"*Live As If* is a beautiful, moving tribute to a woman who truly made this world a better place. Certainly, her legacy as an educator alone is worthy of a story, but Frye Gaillard's portrait of his wife offers so much more; Nancy Gaillard stands as a shining example of grace, courage and generosity. This is a lovely remembrance of a beautiful soul."

—Jill McCorkle, author of *Life After Life* and *Hieroglyphics*; winner of the John Dos Passos Prize for Excellence in Literature

"Nancy Gaillard found much of her meaning in giving—as a teacher, as a friend, in all her relationships. This tribute by her husband, writer Frye Gaillard, is as straightforward, unpretentious, and loving as its subject. It is a story of a life cheerfully and doggedly lived for that which is best in all of us, for hope. It could not be a timelier gift."

—Mike Letcher, Emmy-winning director, Dragonfly Public Media

"Nancy Gaillard was educator extraordinaire, with a passion for learning and a gift for teaching. Nancy's commitment to her profession was evident throughout her career—as a teacher, inspiring young children; as an administrator, mentoring colleagues; and as an instructor, teaching future teachers. She left a treasured legacy that will continue to impact countless lives."

—Andrea Moore Kent, Dean of the College of Education and Professional Studies, University of South Alabama

"Nancy Gaillard's life and work were full of gratitude, love and joy. Those us who knew her followed her final journey with concern and prayers, and in return we were blessed by Nancy's inspiring optimism, her profound insight, her concern for others and her great hope."

—Dr. Stephen Dill, author of *The Poetry of Faith*

"Both intimate and expansive, *Live As If* is a tender and moving portrait of an inspiring teacher, a vibrant and nurturing marriage, and love steadfast against illness and loss. Frye Gaillard's life journey with Nancy, until her passing in 2018, takes us from Charlotte, N.C., during the desegregation of the 1970s, through the backsliding "re-segregation" of the 1990s, to the education department of University of South Alabama in Mobile, where Nancy, forever committed to "reaching every child," mentored a new generation for the classroom. The author, a celebrated journalist, puts facts in the background, though, and speaks from the heart, "love," as he writes, being the "perfect lens" to tell this poignant and uplifting story."

    —Roy Hoffman, winner of the Lillian Smith Book Award, author of the nonfiction *Alabama Afternoons*, and the novels *Come Landfall* and *Chicken Dreaming Corn*

"Frye Gaillard bestows on readers the best gift a book can give, the illusion that we all knew Nancy Gaillard ("Mrs. Schoolyard") as intimately as her family, friends, colleagues, and students did. He has also written an instruction manual: how to live, knowing that (Nancy's words) "little things matter." Little things, like empathy, courage, love of adventure. I read this book in one sitting. It's that graceful, sincere, and endearing. In fact, *Life As If* does the almost impossible; it manages to be heartbreaking and life affirming, both."

    —Judy Goldman, winner of the Sir Walter Raleigh fiction award, author of *Together: A Memoir of a Marriage and a Medical Mishap*

Live as if...

A teacher's love story

written by

Frye Gaillard

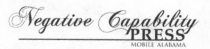
Negative Capability PRESS
MOBILE ALABAMA

Live As If: A teacher's love story

Book and Cover Design by Jenni Krchak
About the cover: Tracy Gaillard Pendergast framed and
photographed the images that comprise the cover art.
Photograph of the grazing horses by Frye Gaillard.
Photograph of Frye and Nancy Gaillard by Paige Vitulli.
Portrait of Nancy taken by Rachel Smook.

ISBN 978-1-7345902-1-0
Library of Congress Control Number: 2020948942

Negative Capability Press
150 Du Rhu Drive, #2202
Mobile, Alabama 36608
(251)591-2922
www.negativecapabilitypress.org
facebook.com/negativecapabilitypress

To all the teachers…

Contents

Foreword

In the prologue to this moving new book about his wife—who died of leukemia in 2018—Frye Gaillard states that "...love is the perfect lens through which to see the story." He's abundantly on target, but it's clear, as well, that Gaillard channels that same love into every sentence he writes, while keeping sentimentality at bay—a feat in itself.

This "story of a teacher" is not just about any teacher, but about *that teacher* (and we've all had them) who one day waves her magic wand over you and a secret portal into a hidden world—of wild surmise and electrifying possibility—swings open and, with a smile, she dares you to walk through it. And there, on the other side, awaits the self you've always longed for, that had existed all along, but your teacher (Nancy Gaillard) had spied it long before you knew it existed—*that teacher* who nurtured dreams for you before you could dream for yourself.

In this harrowing time of Covid-19, when teachers have never been more challenged—often devalued, underpaid, and occasionally demonized—the question remains: Where would we be without them, without Nancy Gaillard, and all the fire-breathing teachers she represents?

Live As If is an unabashed love story—on so many fronts—and how that love, when modeled and embodied fearlessly in a classroom, is ultimately about the Spirit moving in indisputably miraculous ways.

—Joseph Bathanti, former Poet Laureate of North Carolina

Prologue

This is the story of my wife Nancy Gaillard, who died of leukemia on July 27, 2018. Nancy was an educator—classroom teacher, principal, professor—and at every stop on the ladder of her career she did her job about as well as any mortal could. I am biased when I say this, of course. I loved Nancy from the very depths of my heart. But in this case, I think, love is the perfect lens through which to see the story. It was the quality Nancy brought to every part of her life—love of family and friends, love for the work she did as a teacher, love of children of every age, race and class; love of small animals, especially the strays; a love of life in all its possibilities.

Her favorite quote, which she shared below the signature on her emails, came from Gandhi: "Live as if you were to die tomorrow. Learn as if you were to live forever."

For all of her life, even during her time with leukemia, she did her best to live by that advice. So this, unashamedly, is a love story. But it is also the story of education in the midst of social change—of an educator whose career took her through some of the challenges and storms that shaped the latter half of the twentieth century and the early years of the twenty-first. Against the backdrop of racial integration, and sometimes a concerted attack on the efficacies of public education, Nancy set out to make school a place where children would want to come; a place where they could learn.

I have written a lot about education over the course of my career, and this is a story of what can go right. I dedicate it, as Nancy would want, to the teachers out there on the front lines who are doing work that too often goes unappreciated. But this is also the story of Nancy: her work, her life, her legacy. It is also, inevitably, the story of a final journey with leukemia, and the courage and wisdom with which it was lived.

In the last days Rachel, her stepdaughter, told her: "You're still teaching me."

"I always will," Nancy replied. And she said it with a smile.

—Frye Gaillard
University of South Alabama, 2020

PART I: *The Story*

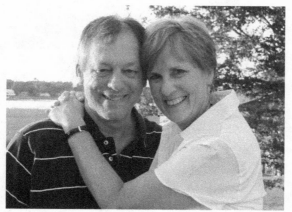

Photo by Carrie Wagner

The Teacher

On the night she died, the two of us lay together in the bed, her hand cradled in the crook of my arm, and knowing that the end was near she looked over at me and smiled. "I'm so happy," she said.

In the nearly two years that have passed since then, I have thought often about that moment. I wish I could say that I shared her optimism and strength, but I did not. Not on that night, nor for most of our thirty-year marriage or the five years of loving friendship that preceded it. For whatever morose combination of reasons, I saw too clearly and felt too keenly the suffering in the world that seemed to define the heart and essence of the human condition.

I knew Nancy Gaillard saw it too. In her final months, she grieved the cruelties of Donald Trump far more openly than she did her own illness, and wondered with her more pessimistic husband at the growing power of our national mean streak. But Nancy's ultimate response to such things was simply to do what she could to embody the opposite.

At that, she was extraordinarily successful—a fact that was readily apparent from the very first moment I met her. She was a third-grade teacher back in those days, working at a magnet school in Charlotte, North Carolina. This was no ordinary school. On September 4, 1957, during its earlier incarnation as a high school, a 15-year-old African-American girl named Dorothy Counts, her face serene and head held high, made her way through a jeering white mob, becoming one of four black students to break the color barrier in Charlotte that day.

It was an ugly moment in the life of that city, a foreshadowing of the turbulence that would soon grip the country as we were confronted, at last, with the sins of our past. But the heroism was apparent also. Kays Gary, one of the great newspaper columnists in the history of the South, wrote about Dorothy in the *Charlotte Observer*. "How many of us," he wondered, "could have taken that walk?"

Don Sturkey, a photographer at that same newspaper, captured an image of Dorothy and the mob of students—hatred twisting the young white faces—that soon made its way around the world. The African-American writer, James Baldwin, living in self-imposed exile, first saw the photograph in a newspaper in Paris. Baldwin had come of age in Harlem, tormented by a stepfather's cruelty and the vast and inescapable racism that, as he understood it, crippled the American heart and soul.

At the age of twenty-four Baldwin left, seeking sanctuary in Paris as other great writers had done—Ernest Hemingway, Richard Wright—but he found that he carried the bitterness with him. "I was forced to admit," he wrote, "something I had always hidden from myself, which the American Negro has been forced to hide from himself as the price of his public progress: that I hated and feared white people…. In effect, I hated and feared the world."

But now, a girl in Charlotte had brought him up short, for here was Dorothy in her innocence and youth, no trace of anger anywhere in her face, no hint of fear in her soft, pretty eyes, confronting the realities from which he had fled. "It made me furious," he wrote. "It filled me with both hatred and pity, and it made me ashamed… It was on that bright afternoon that I knew that I was leaving France."

Soon, he paid his first visit to the South—to the city of Charlotte, where he had discovered, unexpectedly, a face for the hope that he had never felt. In the process, he took his place in the journey toward justice that soon became known as the civil rights movement.

Meanwhile, this school in Charlotte at the center of the storm continued, quietly, to play a pivotal role. Fifteen years later, Harding High School, to which Dorothy had been assigned, had become Irwin Avenue Open Elementary, a magnet school in the inner city, as Charlotte grappled with court-ordered busing. The city had found itself in a social upheaval unlike any in its recent history. In 1971, it became the national test case for busing, and after a unanimous U.S. Supreme Court ruling, racial integration began on a scale for which the community was simply unprepared.

The backlash was immediate and bitter. Mobs of white protesters regularly besieged the school system's headquarters. Racial fighting closed every high school in the system. U.S. District Judge James McMillan, who first ordered busing, was hanged in effigy, and the offices of Julius Chambers, the civil rights lawyer in the case, were burned to the ground.

At Irwin Avenue Open Elementary, the innovative principal, Deane Crowell, hoped her school might be an antidote to the violence. She believed if Irwin, along with other schools, could demonstrate that integration worked, calm in the community might be restored. She had no doubt that this could be done, and buoyed by that article of faith, she assembled a staff of bright young teachers—most of them idealists like herself, who simply loved children, no matter their race or class or circumstances in life.

Nancy Gaillard was one of these teachers. She was Nancy Frederick then, the twenty-five-old wife of a philosophy professor in Charlotte. In 1973, when she took her place on the Irwin Avenue faculty, she came from a school in rural Georgia, where the principal doubled as a Southern Baptist preacher. Once at that school, a little girl fell on the playground and broke her arm, an injury so serious that the jagged end of a bone had made an ugly tear in the skin.

The principal's response was stern. "Jesus won't love you if you cry," he said.

Nancy took the little girl in her arms. "Cry all you want, Sweetheart," she replied.

She told me that story in one of our earliest conversations. All her life, she explained, she found that schools were all too often forbidding places for a young person to be. Early on in Charlotte, when she was a third-grader at Merry Oaks Elementary, many of her peers—at her instigation—began calling their school

Sad Pines Penitentiary. Nancy was certain that she could do better.

At Irwin Avenue she reveled in the chance.

I met her briefly during those beginning days of her career. As the education reporter for the *Charlotte Observer*, I was doing a story on Irwin Avenue and Nancy was one of the teachers I interviewed. Years later, I would remember the sparkle in her eyes as she talked about the children in her class—black and white, and the Hmong refugees from the highlands of Laos. But I don't remember that Nancy stood out from the rest—from colleagues like Carolyn Coffey and Steve Houser, committed, hard-working educators who were also two of her close friends.

Together, they embraced the freewheeling philosophy of their principal, arranging their classes in multiage groups, creating their own instructional materials to meet the needs of individual children, and working most often with small groups of students who helped in the planning of their own education. They also embraced their inner city home. One startling morning they arrived at the school to find a dead man lying on the steps. He was homeless and had simply expired in the lonely chill of the preceding night. All they could do was call the authorities and remove the body before the children got there.

That was life in the inner city. But as Carolyn Coffey remembers, there was a richness about it also. "There was a cemetery," she recalled, "out behind the school, and we would take the children to do grave rubbings. We took them up town to the St. Patrick's Day parade. We had fun with the kids. We did crazy things."

One of the craziest came on January 20, 1981. Carolyn

and Nancy decided to take their class of forty-five students—a combination of third, fourth and fifth graders—plus another five students with behavioral problems, to the presidential inauguration in Washington. There were fifty children in all, ages eight through ten, including some of the most unruly in the school. Many had never been out of Charlotte, much less imagined the pomp and ceremony of the nation's peaceful transfer of power.

In the lead up to what Principal Deane Crowell called "this mother of all field trips," the teachers taught lessons on civics and geography, and recruited parents and teacher aides to go along as chaperones. Each adult was assigned three or four students.

On January 20, a mild winter morning (the inauguration temperature was 55 degrees), they boarded a train at 3:30 a.m. At the last minute one student panicked, insisting that he didn't want to go just as the train was about to leave the station. "We did a little fast talking," Carolyn said, and the boy relented.

They made it to the Capitol late in the morning, and a few of the students were able to see the presidential limousine as it passed. All of them posed on the Capitol steps with their own representative in Congress. They also witnessed a moment in history—a spectacle repeated every four years since April 20, 1789, when George Washington took his first oath of office.

Then it was over. At 4 p.m., they re-boarded the train for the eight-hour trip back to Charlotte. "A long day," Carolyn remembered. It was also an audacious excursion that somehow went off without a hitch. Nancy often talked about it with a smile. "Amazingly," she said, "we did not lose a single child."

Such was the atmosphere at Irwin Avenue, where Deane Crowell and her successors, Bruce Irons and Mildred Wright, encouraged the boldness of their bright young staff, pushed them to ask "what if?" and "why not?" instead of settling for the status quo. Steve Houser remembered how they started a summer enrichment program for inner city students—children who needed something to do in neighborhoods that were often riddled with crime.

He and Nancy decided to meet every morning in the heart of downtown—at the commercial crossroads of Trade and Tryon Streets—and venture forth with the students to see what the city had to offer. One hot summer day, they set out for an area called Optimist Park, a neighborhood not far away, where Jimmy Carter was building houses for Habitat for Humanity. "For safety reasons," said Houser, "we couldn't actually work on the construction of these houses with the adult workers, so we went to a small church that was next door and did service work by weeding their community garden. President Carter and Rosalynn walked over and thanked the children for their service to this neighborhood. I can assure you that those children never forgot that day. Nancy and I never forgot it either."

Later, when we became friends, Nancy would talk about those times, about her daily astonishment at feeling so free to do what she thought was right for her students. She said she sometimes channeled her heroes—people like Jonathan Kozol, who wrote in *Death at an Early Age* about his experience as a teacher in the inner city of Boston; or Mister Rogers, a friend of Kozol's who became an icon—almost an educational saint—because of his infectious love of little kids. And finally, most colorfully, she kept a dog-eared copy of *The Water Is Wide*, the first bestseller by Pat Conroy, who wrote about the children of Daufuskie Island, where he had taken a one-year job as a teacher.

Daufuskie, a barrier island off the coast of South Carolina, unconnected to the mainland by a bridge, was a place of extraordinary isolation. Even as late as the 1970s, ox carts rumbled down its sandy lanes, where the marsh gave way to live oak forests, and snake-friendly thickets of palmetto and briars surrounded little clusters of unpainted shacks. Many of the children who lived in this place were so cut off from the outside world that they did not know the name of their country.

On his first day on the island, Conroy asked the students in his class, grades five through eight, to write a brief paragraph about themselves. Bewildered stares greeted this request. Conroy gamely repeated the assignment, and in *The Water Is Wide*, he wrote about what happened next:

As I walked around my new fiefdom, the kids earnestly applying themselves to the task at hand, I had my first moment of panic. Some of them could barely write. Half of them were incapable of expressing even the simplest thought on paper. Three quarters of them could barely spell even the most elementary words. Three of them could not write their names. Sweet little Jesus, I thought, as I weaved between the desks, these kids don't know crap.

Nancy would laugh when she quoted that passage. But it was a serious reminder of a fundamental truth—the duty of a teacher to meet her students where they were, no matter the limitations they brought to the class, and figure out how to move forward together. At Irwin Avenue, the challenges were generally less acute than the ones Conroy encountered on the island. But not always. The children of Hmong refugees, who had survived the killing fields of Asia, often came to school without a single word of English.

But it was not just those from war torn places, the ones who lived with hunger, or struggled with the deprivations of poverty. Many years later a middle class student, Carolyn Edsall-Vetter, would remember a life-changing moment in Nancy's kindergarten class. "I was an early reader," she said, "and used to balk at napping. Nancy let me put my mat down by the bookcase and the bright window so I could read instead of sleeping. It might not seem like a big thing, but in contrast to other teachers who put 'the rules' over intellectual and emotional learning, Nancy's willingness to negotiate with me around my interests, learning style, and personality taught me that my ideas had value, that I could—and must—advocate for myself, and that school was a place to learn, not just to 'behave.' I think this message was particularly important for her as a woman to be teaching and modeling for young girls." Carolyn also remembered that Nancy taught her class in sneakers and jeans. "She was just so down to earth and real."

In Nancy's own recollections about Irwin Avenue, there was another student who stood out from the rest. Not that she wanted to put it that way, for every child was precious. Still, there was something special about Christian Elmore. He was a bright little boy who came from an upper middle class family, but had a hard time learning to read. Nancy became his tutor. They met together two or three times a week for the rest of his time at Irwin, and a bit less often all the way to high school.

"Nancy was an awesome person," Christian would remember. Sometimes she would help him with homework. Other times they would play memory games, with playing cards face down on the floor where the two of them were sitting. And she taught him chess, with all the mental exercise it required. "I still play," he says.

For the most part, as the weeks of tutoring stretched into months, and then into years, there were no Miracle Worker moments—no magical breakthroughs—just a lot of hard work and patience, as Christian gradually learned to work around his initial difficulties with reading. Nancy knew he was not alone. The mind of every child, even the brightest, had its own wiring, and she never doubted that Christian would succeed. And of course he did.

When he earned an engineering degree from North Carolina State University, his mother, Maria Elmore, wrote Nancy a letter: "I am sure Christian is only one of many you have helped as a result of your great love and skills. We will never forget what you did for us all."

For teachers like Nancy, or Carolyn Coffey and Steve Houser, this was always the heart of the mission: finding a way to reach every child, and success was measured in the lives of their students. But in Charlotte there was another dimension to the story, a metanarrative that went with the daily pressures of teaching. In this politically charged era of desegregation, the responsibility fell on principals and teachers to knit together a diverse student body. Together they had made the great leap of faith, later confirmed in educational studies, that this was really the best way to do it—that children of every race and class learn most effectively in a real-world setting, a microcosm of the community around them.

They could see from headlines out of Boston and Detroit, and other school districts around the country, that the nation as a whole was resisting this notion. But in Charlotte, after a rocky start, this journey of faith caught the public imagination and began to reshape the life of the community. Charlotte, more than most American cities, was working to come to terms with its past—to build a future that would be more just. And the work of teachers lay at the heart of the struggle.

The Principal

In the spring of 1983, I was still writing about such things when Nancy and I became friends. We discovered that we were neighbors. She was married to Norris, the philosophy professor, and I was living as a bachelor around the corner, sharing rent with a sportswriter from the *Charlotte Observer*. In those days, which are now a blur, the women who wandered into my life came to know I was not a good bet. My first marriage had ended with a lot of pain, almost all of it caused by me, and I was not eager to repeat the mistake.

Girlfriends came and girlfriends went. One was a bank teller who worked downtown, a beautiful young woman who took pride in her Cherokee ancestry. Another was a grad student in Chapel Hill, working on her doctorate in political science. She especially deserved a better fate. But I was battling demons from an earlier time, and good women came to know the dark side well—the terrified boy I kept hidden away, who only Nancy seemed to know how to soothe. Maybe it was because she was married and I found her safe. Whatever it was, the two of us discovered we could talk in a way that, for both of us, was new.

At first we talked about the schools. Charlotte, we agreed, was a unique place, where some of the most affluent leaders in the city had cast their lot with the public schools. There was a sense of civic pride that was hard to explain—eloquent ministers who preached on Sundays about the necessity of integration; businessmen who seemed to understand the promise as well as the burdens of change; and black leaders deeply committed to the schools. This was how it seemed to us, and we were delighted, each in our way, to be a part of something so grand.

Gradually, our conversations became more personal, and we also talked about our lives. Nancy said she had married young, and she and her husband, good man that he was, were beginning to find the road more rocky. She said they wanted different things out of life. I, meanwhile, continued to fail at every relationship I began. Even after three years of therapy, I was beginning to assume this was how it would be, when everything changed. Nancy's marriage ended, and within a year her husband remarried and she and I were falling in love.

It felt like the culmination of a friendship.

Three years of glorious courtship followed, enriched by travel to fascinating places—Yellowstone and the Black Hills of South Dakota, the Bahamas, Jamaica and the Soviet Union; the city of Baku on the Caspian Sea. On that latter stop, in what was soon to become the independent nation of Azerbaijan, we walked together down medieval streets and ate meals from menus we could not read. We also found a restive population—mostly

Muslim—chafing at Soviet control of their country.

One bright morning as we were walking, we came to a building our tourist guide had pointed out the day before. It was the headquarters, drab and forbidding, of the Muslim radicals who were trying to overthrow the Russians.

"Let's go in," Nancy said.

"What?" I replied, thinking I must have misunderstood. "You want to go inside?"

"Sure," she said. "Maybe we can learn about what's going on."

I found myself, as I would on other occasions with Nancy, torn between my instinct for caution and an impulse common among my half of the species. I did not wish to be seen as a wimp. "Okay," I said.

Utter silence greeted our entry, as a group of armed men regarded us, not so much with hostility, it seemed, as with pure astonishment that we were there. Finally, they led us to a room upstairs, and with one of them standing guard at the door, another began to ask us questions. We did not, of course, understand a word he was saying. Nor did he understand our replies, as I tried to explain with a facsimile of calm that we were tourists from the United States—teachers, I said, (a journalist, I thought, might arouse more suspicion) who wanted to learn about their place.

After a while of mounting frustration, the two men left us sitting there alone, their gestures making clear that we could not leave. We waited for an hour or more, a time, we agreed, that was passing very slowly. "Well," I said, trying to keep our spirits up, "this will make a great story if we survive."

Another man came in eventually, a speaker of badly broken English, who carried himself with an air of command. He was stern at first, though he did not seem especially hostile, and after another round of questions, he told us we could go. These two Americans, he had clearly decided, were far too stupid to pose any threat. "Go back to your hotel," he said.

We did as we were told, and waited there until hunger overtook us. As dusk was settling over Baku, and the sounds of the city drifted in from the streets, we ventured to a restaurant just down the block. We ordered another delicious meal, again from a menu we could not read.

This was how it was with Nancy, as we began our journey of adventure together, laughing all the way. In 1988, we married, and I was more in love than I thought I could be. But these were also restless times. I had grown weary of newspaper work—the daily deadlines, the bosses with whom I did not get along—and I decided to leave the *Charlotte Observer* to become a full-time writer of books. It was a perilous economic decision, but Nancy was all in. She pointed out that she was earning a steady paycheck, and she was sure everything would be fine. Besides, she said, she was also ready for a change. She was eager now to pursue an ambition that she had nursed since she was a child. She wanted to run her own school.

With a good bit of sadness, she left the classroom and applied to become an Assistant Principal. By the early 1990s, after a brief apprenticeship, she found herself assigned to a school that was everything she had ever hoped for. She became the new principal at Billingsville Elementary, a public Montessori school in the inner city.

Like Irwin Avenue, Billingsville was a place with a rich and inspirational history. It began its life as a Rosenwald School, part of the philanthropic dream of Booker T. Washington and a Jewish millionaire named Julius Rosenwald. Together, they decided in 1913 to build schools for black children all over the South. With Rosenwald providing the seed money, they built 5,000 schools in the next twenty years, changing the face of public education in one of the poorest parts of America.

Rosenwald came to this project as the CEO of Sears Roebuck. Under his leadership Sears had become the Amazon of its day, relying on catalogues more than freestanding stores to expand its reach to every corner of the country. As the profits rolled in and he became a rich man, Rosenwald began to consider what to do with his wealth. In 1910, one of his friends, Paul Sachs, a founding partner of Goldman Sachs, and a supporter of the NAACP, gave him a copy of *Up from Slavery*, Booker T. Washington's autobiography. As soon as he finished reading the book, Rosenwald decided to pay a visit to this great man, who served as president of Tuskegee Institute in the rural backwaters of Alabama.

Almost without exception, the schools they began to build together became the objects of community pride. Certainly, this was true of Billingsville, which took its name from Sam Billings, the farmer who provided the land. Mr. Billings and his neighbors, who were African American, regarded their school—which they had physically helped to build—as a shining symbol of progress.

Nancy knew this history well, and understood clearly that it was a strength on which she could build. But she knew that this was a delicate assignment. Billingsville was a magnet school, and its mission in the days of integration was to entice white parents in the wealthy suburbs to send their children to school in the city—to a neighborhood that was nearly all black. Generally, this worked well, thanks in part to the vision of Maria Montessori.

Dr. Montessori was a physician, born in Italy in 1870, and one of the first women in her country to enter this profession. She was especially interested in psychiatry, and nursed a corollary fascination with children and the way they learned. In 1907, she opened a child-care program in one of the poorest neighborhoods in Rome. The children at first were an unruly group, whose parents often left them to fend for themselves, as mothers and fathers worked at hardscrabble jobs, trying desperately to make ends meet. Many observers thought such children were hopeless. Dr. Montessori did not.

She gave them puzzles and other materials to engage their interest, taught them to garden and cook, and after a while she noticed that they were teaching themselves. Over the years she refined her technique, and the Montessori method became an international educational movement. Most of the teachers in Nancy's school believed in it deeply.

"This philosophy," explained Dryw Freed, who taught third grade, "was based on an enduring respect for children as people. Dr. Montessori's main goals were to teach children independence and introduce them to the beauty of the natural world and the wonders of science."

At Billingsville that was the plan, but there was also a problem. In the 1990s, the reality that hovered over public education was an obsession with standardized test scores as a measure of whether a school was succeeding. For a subject like math, or even reading, the Montessori method was different from the kind of linear instruction that translated easily to a test. The first year's scores were disappointing. Soon, word came down from the central office that improvements had to come quickly, or else.

Freed said Nancy sheltered her staff from that pressure: "She said she would take the heat." But patiently, other teachers remembered, Nancy persuaded them to make subtle changes. Some students simply needed a more structured approach, and in a series of staff meetings and workshops, they talked at length—teachers free to speak their minds—about how they could modify the Montessori method, holding to the heart of the philosophy, to meet the needs of every child. One teacher, Beth Leo, described Nancy's leadership in that time as "kind, giving, loving, and supportive."

I would listen to such assessments and know they were true. But I knew there was another dimension as well. "Nancy was a force of nature in achieving goals," said her friend, Lynn Smith-Loving, a sociologist at Duke University, who talked often with her about their work. And Sherri Faulk, her assistant principal, added: "She was the epitome of a good listener. She also had a way of leading people to do the things she wanted them to do—things that made them better."

Whatever the reason, test scores rose in the second year. Pressure from the central office abated, and applications soared from parents who wanted their children in the school. There was, however, another challenge more daunting than the first. There were parts of Grier

Heights, the neighborhood around Billingsville, where the crime rate was high, and drug dealers gathered at dusk on the corners, and even the good people were afraid.

One afternoon a little girl who lived in Grier Heights came to the principal's office in tears. "Mrs. Gaillard," she said, "I missed my bus and I'm afraid to walk home by myself."

"I'll walk with you, Sweetheart," Nancy replied, and the two of them set out together for a house that proved to be a mile away. It was a trek full of cheerful conversation, but the sun was sinking low in the sky when Nancy began the long walk back. The drug dealers and their customers had begun to gather. "Hey, guys," said Nancy, as she approached a group of men. "I need you to help me take care of my school."

A few of them stared back with hard eyes, while others grew sullen and turned away. But after a moment one of them said, "Okay, ma'am, we'll try."

Nancy's friend, Ted Fillette, a Legal Aid lawyer whose work took him often to Grier Heights, would later marvel at that encounter, and how the word went out in the neighborhood that this white lady was not afraid.

"She accosted the leading drug dealer in the area," said Fillette, "and asked him to protect the school so that she could get the Grier Heights kids what they needed. That was fearless and showed a selfless disregard for her personal security. But, it also showed an uncommon wisdom. She must have thought that this drug dealer was once a child and probably did not get his needs met. She knew that even a drug dealer wants to feel good about himself and could take some civic pride in helping the underserved kids in Grier Heights get what he missed. That is real wisdom. That is focused determination to succeed in a tough environment."

Things, of course, did not change overnight. One afternoon about the same time, Nancy and Sherrie Faulk, were talking together in her office when they heard a pinging sound, then cracking glass, on the window just above them. They rushed outside and saw a grinning sixth grader on his bike, pellet gun in hand. Before the boy could escape Sherrie had a grip on his handlebars, and she and Nancy took him home to see his grandmother.

"She took away the pellet gun," remembered Sherrie, "and said we would not have any more trouble. We always got along well with the grandparents."

In the aftermath of this adventure, Sherrie and Nancy launched an afterschool program—a Boys Club for some of the most notorious troublemakers, complete with a basketball team for those who behaved. They practiced at the original Rosenwald school, now a community center on the edge of the campus, and participation was strictly conditional. No vandalism. No fighting. Homework assignments turned in on time.

In addition to the athletic competition, they began a music program with instruments provided through a local business, and one of the toughest boys in the club showed an aptitude for the violin. "But I can't take it home to practice," he said. Other boys, he explained, would make fun of him and might even smash the instrument to bits. They found him a room to practice at school.

And so it went day after day, as Nancy and her staff worked to make school a happy destination. Every morning she greeted the children as they came through the door, calling their names, giving them hugs, and progress was tangible as well as anecdotal. As test scores rose, and applications soared, with the help of community policemen—specially trained officers who worked closely with the school—the crime rate in Grier Heights fell.

As the years went by, Sherri Faulk noticed something else as well. "We had fun," she said. It was one of their takeaways—one of the contagious feelings among teachers and students that emanated partly from the principal's office. I know for sure that Nancy felt it. I could see it in her face, and hear it in her stories, almost every night when she came home. I remember her particular moment of pride on the day she learned that her school—alone among more than a hundred in the system—had reached its yearly attendance goals. When an administrator asked her how they had done it, Nancy said it was simple: "We try to make this a place where children want to come."

There was satisfaction in that, but there were also storm clouds on the horizon. In the growing city of Charlotte, many of the new citizens were skeptical of the notion of integration. They came most often from the North or Midwest, where the suburban schools they were accustomed to were more homogenous than those in Charlotte. A group of parents took the school district to court, and in 1999 a conservative federal judge ruled that race could not be a factor in the way that children were assigned to their schools. On the surface this sounded color blind. But what it meant in practice was that the school system could no longer pursue an intentional policy of integration.

In the rapid re-segregation that followed, racial tensions, ironically, were beginning to return, and Nancy's school was not immune. The problems often came in unexpected disguise. There was one little girl with Down syndrome whose mother wanted her to be mainstreamed—just another child at the school, respected and loved and not set apart, treated like any other student. Nancy was sympathetic to that request. Her own son Chris had a stepbrother with Down syndrome, and there was not a sweeter little boy anywhere. But the child at Nancy's school had a problem. She liked to pull other children's hair. Her grip was strong and she would not let go, and the result was often a handful of hair with bloody roots. To make matters worse, the troubled hair-puller was African American and many of her victims were white, and soon the school had unhappy parents.

Nancy was able to get the problem solved, but not as quickly as she wanted. Regulations and red tape did not make it easy. It occurred to her around that time that she was getting tired, and early in the fall of 2003, she confessed these feelings to Debra Davis, one of her most trusted teachers.

"Nancy was a friend and an incredible educator," said Davis. "But I think in time her ability and willingness to work with parents, her patience in listening, made her somewhat weary. We were sitting in her office talking and she mentioned that she had put in the paperwork to retire. Although I knew the time might be coming, it was still an emotional moment for me. When she later announced her retirement at a staff meeting, I cried—and I am not a big crier—as though it was the first time I heard it."

On her final day, a teacher gave Nancy a packet of notes composed by students. "We love you, Mrs. Schoolyard," wrote one little girl, who had never managed to get the name right. Nancy was delighted by this particular mangling, choosing not to correct it, and she laughed again as she showed me the note.

At the end of one chapter, and the beginning of another, this was all she needed to know.

The Professor

During the first fifteen years of our marriage, we had lived on a horse farm outside of Charlotte. "Horse farm" probably overstates the case. We owned five acres, one of which was wooded with a cedar farmhouse nestled in the trees. A rambling porch stretched across the front, and beyond the trees, horses grazed in a four-acre pasture, rolling gently down toward a pond. Some of the horses came and went, but two of them became a permanent part of the family.

Nancy had never been around horses, but I had reveled in their company during boyhood summers on my uncle's farm. I had always dreamed of owning my own, and Nancy, not surprisingly, thought this sounded like a grand idea. Her favorite of our two gentle beasts was Hoodie—whose name, we learned, was short for Houdini because of her skill at opening gates. We would find her some mornings grazing happily in the yard, the grass being greener just beyond her fence. We would lead her patiently back to the pasture, and do our best to improve on the locks.

I used to say that life would be fine, as long as I did not outlive Hoodie. The bond between Nancy and this handsome quarter horse, who was going on eighteen when we bought her, was a tender and remarkable thing to behold. At the sight of Nancy, Hoodie would nicker and amble toward the barn, hoping for food and a little bit of grooming. She weighed almost a thousand pounds, but in Nancy's presence had the disposition of a kitten.

We tried not to think about the fact that she was getting old. She didn't act like it, and obviously found great contentment in the company of Nancy—and even more, her pasture-mate T, a high-stepping Morgan whose original name had been T-Bird. T was a stylish, intelligent horse, well trained and obedient, but ready to run anytime a grownup set foot in the stirrups. But with a child as a passenger, T would drop her head and knew instinctively, sweetly that this was a cargo to be treated with care. She and Hoodie were inseparable, and for more than a decade, on long trail rides back through the woods, they brought great joy to the humans in the family.

But time does pass and horses get old, and eventually, sadly enough, they die. Hoodie went first. At the age of 32, she simply expired. T lived another year, grieving inconsolably until the end. She would stand alone in the pasture, sometimes not even bothering to graze, as her head drooped low in the afternoon sun. It was a heart-breaking thing to see, and no amount of attention—not even another horse we bought for her as company—seemed to offer much consolation.

When T died too, having become so lame she could barely walk, we felt like an era had come to an end.

Nancy had just retired, and we began to talk about moving to the coast of Alabama. I had grown up there, and
my mother, who lived in my childhood home, was now
pushing ninety. Her health was visibly beginning to fail,
and I was an only child. There was nobody else to take
care of her.

About that time, I received an offer to be writer in
residence at the University of South Alabama, and it
seemed clear enough that the stars had aligned. In place
of the horses, we bought a house on the water, on a tidal
river just south of Mobile, where ospreys nested in the
cypress trees and Great Blue Herons waded in the marsh.
We bought a little boat for exploring the river, and every
morning for the next fifteen years—and I am not exag-
gerating when I say this—Nancy would gaze out the
window and marvel at the fact that this was where we
lived.

Such was her love of beauty and life and the adventures that came with a brand new place. She discovered
that she was much too restless to retire. For the past
several years, she had nurtured a couple of bucket list
ambitions, the first of which was to teach at a college.
She applied for a job at South Alabama's College of Education, and was hired as an adjunct. Her first assignment,
much to her delight, was to mentor student teachers in
the field.

As she began her new mission, she could see again
that a central issue confronting public schools—the larger
reality that teachers were facing—was a variation on the
old theme of integration. They were dealing with a new
diversity; the ranges of ethnicity and race were broad-
er than they had ever been before. Mobile, in that way,

was like many other cities in the country. The student bodies in most of its schools included Latinos, Laotians, and Vietnamese, immigrants from Africa and the Middle East, as well as Americans from poor neighborhoods, including many African Americans. There were white students too, but many of those whose parents could afford it were now attending private schools. They were part of a flood of refugees from public education, raised in families who had come to believe that the public schools did not measure up.

Nancy was certain those families were wrong. She could see there were problems in some schools—most of them a product of too little funding. But there were good things happening as well, teachers working creatively and hard to meet the needs of every child. She was eager for her future teachers to embrace this example. This became her message, her contagious affirmation, and her colleagues at South Alabama quickly noticed.

"With her prior experience as a principal," said Andi Kent, Dean of the College, "she was quite the natural in working with our students. She would nurture and mentor, but could also exhibit tough love, especially when it came to helping the students see the world was bigger than themselves."

Susan Santoli, her department chair, was struck by Nancy's attention to detail. She remembered a visit the two of them made to a low-income school. "As we walked in," Santoli recalled, "Nancy commented about the lack of any outside landscaping or anything that would make a positive first impression. Before long, that school had two large planters, full of plants, outside of the main doors donated anonymously by Nancy." It was a little thing, but little things mattered—a lesson Nancy wanted her students to remember.

At South Alabama, as at other places, her colleagues soon became her friends. "I do not remember the exact day I met Nancy," said Kelly Byrd, whose office was just down the hall. "But I could see from the start the kind of spirit she would bring to our work family. There was never a time that she was not smiling and not encouraging everyone around her—students and faculty the same. She stopped by my office every morning on the way to hers. If I was stressed or struggling with anything, life in general, sometimes, she stayed and talked with me—not concerned about time or anything else but our time together. She always left me with a bit more encouraged to face whatever was coming my way."

Benterah Morton, one of her favorite young professors, added, "I thought she was a witty ray of sunshine." The two of them met when Morton came to the University for a job interview. As an African American, he wondered about the racial climate in a deep Southern city but was not sure how to bring it up. Nancy did it for him. "Benterah," she said, "there are different types of people here in Mobile. We give the other people Mardi Gras and they don't bother us the rest of the year."

Morton smiled. It was a judgment, he thought, delivered with reassuring candor and wit. Yes, there were powerful forces in the community whose priorities could be self-indulgent and shallow—people more interested in pageantry than progress. But it was also possible for people like themselves to make a difference.

"While I was shocked that she would share such candid information with me at this stage," said Morton,

"I was relieved that someone was willing to address the racism in the city. I recall chuckling to myself and thinking, 'This lady is alright with me.'"

For her part, almost from the start, Nancy felt more at home at South Alabama than she had in her final years in Charlotte, where job satisfactions were sometimes clouded by the administrators above her. One superintendent had expressed private doubts that a person as "nice" as Nancy—a term he did not intend as a compliment—could really be an effective principal. As a general rule, she put such annoyances out of her mind, or tried to, but at South Alabama there was no need. She simply fit in.

Nancy found inspiration in the mission of this university—an aspiration that dovetailed powerfully with the purposes of public education. This was, after all, a public university and it was anything but elite. It did not pride itself on the number of applicants it rejected for admission. Half its students were the first in their families to go to college, and many of them came from small rural schools not rich in resources. But in Nancy's experience they were hungry to learn, and the university faculty was hungry to teach them, and all of it was happening at a time of education under siege. In the real world their students would enter, racial diversity was complicated by the national reality of re-segregation, which was a maddening fact of life in Alabama. Inadequate funding was a perennial problem, and with it class size and teacher compensation. And standardized testing was still double-edged—successful perhaps in holding schools accountable, but with the unintended consequence of discouraging teachers from taking risks or pursuing the kind of creative instruction that had shaped her own career.

These were the problems young teachers would face, precisely at a time when the needs of children were becoming more complicated and diverse. Nancy was eager to help them prepare, and the way to do it, she tried to say—on the other side of the bewildering complications of the job—was to keep their focus always on the child.

This was challenge enough for anybody, and for most of her first six years at South, Nancy was happy in her role. She was the utility player. She taught her courses, mentored young teachers, and sometimes pinch-hit for a professor on sabbatical. The stress was low, at least compared to the life of a principal, and it was easy to see she was part of the glue that held things together.

"It was as if," said Karyn Tunks, who had an office down the hall, "she seamlessly became a part of the faculty from the start."

Even as she embraced her job, Nancy found herself, sometime around the seventh year, pondering the last of her own ambitions. This one was personal, something she wanted to do for herself, even if it might seem self-indulgent. She wanted to pursue her Ph.D., beginning this quest at the age of 62.

"It's silly, right?" she would say when we discussed it.

"Not if you really want to do it," I said. "I think it's great."

"Do you think I can do it?"

"Of course you can do it. You can do anything you set your mind to. You don't have to do it. Professionally, you have nothing to prove. But I can see in your eyes you really want to. Besides, if you go to the University of Alabama, maybe you can be a cheerleader."

We laughed a lot about that image—Nancy standing erect, pom-poms in hand, balanced in the palm of a male cheerleader, raising her voice for the Crimson Tide. At the same time, as she was finally making up her mind, I thought seriously about why she wanted to take this on. I know she did too. It was certainly not the promotion from Senior Instructor to Assistant Professor that she thought might come when she completed the task. Nor was it the modest increase in pay. And while she was always eager to learn something new, I'm pretty sure she didn't think she needed a doctorate to be a good teacher. I think it may have started with a wound.

There was a teacher she had, either in elementary or junior high school, who had also taught her sister, Harriett. Harriett was always a high achiever. Later, in the course of her career, she earned her doctorate in physical therapy and an international reputation as a wound care specialist. Nancy and I were both proud of her. But as a child Nancy had been deeply hurt when the teacher she and Harriett shared told her one day: "You are not as brilliant as your sister. What happened to you?"

This was a reminder of the double-edged possibilities of teaching. Teachers could do so much good, but could also inflict such hurt. It was a reason Nancy knew that she could do better.

Over the course of our time together, she talked about this episode enough that I knew the injury went deep. She was a child, after all, when it happened. Despite her radiant optimism and confidence, which were also strong, she was susceptible to occasional slights and doubts that came from people important to her. In the end, however, whatever her private complications,

I think she was mostly driven by the challenge, the new adventure, that would make life richer. In any case, she decided to do it.

For the next five years she commuted back and forth to the University of Alabama—a three and a half hour drive from Mobile—while teaching full-time at South Alabama. In the summer session, she rented a house in Tuscaloosa. She loved her time in this college town— loved the clocks in the restaurants and bars that counted down by the second, beginning in the spring, to the moment of kickoff in September. The football team ("my little boys," she called them, who she would watch on television every Saturday) won three national championships while she was there. She was happy to claim her part of the credit.

But she also worked incredibly hard. Her friend, Robin Harvey, another doctoral student, would remember the morning when the two of them met. They had climbed three flights of marble stairs in the education building, and were sitting on a bench outside the classroom, waiting for the professor to arrive. They began to talk and Robin thought immediately this was somebody special. There was something in the smile and the eyes, she said, something in the quality of the listening that made it clear, The more they talked, the less peculiar it seemed that Nancy was undertaking this challenge at a time in life when most people would not. "It made perfect sense," Robin said. "It was who she was."

They encouraged each other in the coming months, and it was obvious that Nancy had no hesitation about asking friends and family for help. Her husband became the copy editor for her dissertation, tightening sentences and syntax while Nancy pored through federal court cases about the Fourth and Fifth Amendment rights of students. Abigail Baxter, her South Alabama colleague, helped her fact-check and analyze data. On Friday afternoons, she and Kelly Byrd, who was about to begin her own dissertation, would meet in a conference room at the college, articles and papers scattered on a table, each working separately, each holding the other accountable.

Then finally it was done. On May 7, 2016, when Nancy's graduation day arrived, family members descended on Tuscaloosa. Her son Chris, daughter-in-law Jarin, and grandson Lincoln flew in from Durham; Harriett drove up from Thomasville, Georgia, and stepdaughter Tracy and Gemma, the youngest grandchild, flew across the country from Portland. The mood was festive as we gathered that night, lots of family stories and laughter. There was also drinking involved. The following morning, when she crossed the stage in her cap and gown, most of us agreed we had never seen her happier. We thought her smile might split open her face.

On the night after, when we took a deep breath, I told her I needed to clarify the etiquette. "Do I have to call you Dr. Nancy," I asked, "even when it's just the two of us?"

"Well," she replied, "that would be nice." And both of us laughed.

As our conversation moved from silly to tender, as such conversations so often did, we talked about how when she was thirty-five, she ran the Marine Corps Marathon in Washington, D.C. She thought at the time, despite the satisfaction it brought her, that her first marathon would be her last. The doctorate, she said, felt like her second.

It never crossed our minds on this happy occasion that a much harder marathon lay just ahead.

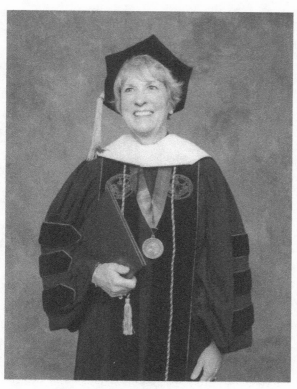

 University of Alabama
Commencement Ceremony   ZAP
May 7, 2016

The Illness

About the time she became Dr. Nancy, a designation quickly adopted by the family (and one she accepted with some delight) I was finishing an opus—*A Hard Rain: America in the 1960s,* which weighed in at 800 manuscript pages. Nancy had read every word and she was happy to report to everybody who would listen that this was going to be the best one yet. Nancy was like that.

In our time of mutual exhaustion, which began in the fall of 2016, both of us discovered a new favorite pastime, which was one we sometimes pursued together: Sleep. I had always been pretty good at it, and Nancy was catching on quickly. Ten-hour nights were not uncommon. At the same time, we began to consider a mutual reward that we might bestow upon one another for our hard work.

These ruminations turned naturally to travel. Nancy had been to many places—Scandinavia and Greece with her teacher-friends, India and Dubai with her sister. She had also discovered that because of assignments that went with my job, I was close to having visited all fifty states. She eagerly embraced this challenge, even when the destinations were North Dakota or Iowa. (In the former, we communed with wild mustangs in Theodore Roosevelt National Park. We were not disappointed.)

In 2017, we began to talk about Africa. I had been there once, and Nancy loved the photographs from Uganda—wild elephants and hippos and crocodiles lazing on the banks of a river. She was intrigued by a feeling I had found overwhelming when my plane first touched down in Entebbe. I had the sense that I had been there before. Imagination can play its tricks, but I would have sworn this was coming from my DNA. Nancy wanted to see for herself.

We made an appointment with a travel agent, but before we could keep it something happened during one of her classes. On an afternoon in April, she became weak and nauseous and had to end the session early. One of her colleagues called and I came immediately and found her sweaty and pale and draped in a chair. I rushed her to the emergency room, where she was admitted with cardiac arrhythmia—an irregular heartbeat, the doctor explained, though he was not sure of the cause.

As we awaited more tests, my mind flashed back to a dark premonition from a few months earlier when Nancy and Norris, her ex-husband who had remained a good friend, went to visit a high school classmate who was dying from a brain tumor. David McKnight was a brilliant writer and musician, who had struggled in his life with mental illness, and earned a living in his later years playing his fiddle on a street corner in Durham. He played it beautifully. As Nancy was telling me about the visit—she said David was happy they had come—a shadow of dread passed across my mind: What if something happened to Nancy? It was a thought quickly banished, for it made no sense. She had always been healthy. I was the one with diabetes and high blood pressure, and we laughed sometimes about the handful of pills I took every day. "Just doing my part for big pharma," I said.

At the ER that night, after a long wait, there was no real diagnosis of the problem. The doctor gave her medication for the symptoms and suggested she see a cardiologist. As we left the hospital, neither of us was especially worried. She continued, however, to have issues with fatigue, and while her heart doctors tinkered with the medication, we decided to postpone the trip to Africa. We went to New Mexico instead to celebrate her birthday in the rugged highlands north of Santa Fe.

In the thin mountain air, she was often short of breath, becoming winded on the short walk from our room at the lodge to the parking lot. More tests followed when we returned to Mobile. The cardiologist discovered she was anemic. Seriously anemic. She needed an immediate blood transfusion. They did a bone marrow biopsy and discovered leukemia. And not just *any* leukemia. This was AML—Acute Myeloid Leukemia—in which the bone marrow goes haywire and produces blasts: fat and bloated red blood cells that do nothing worthwhile and simply take up space. Of the eight or so forms of AML, hers was the worst and most difficult to treat.

We made arrangements to go MD Anderson in Houston, the most renowned leukemia center in the world. Her appointment was for August 28. Hurricane Harvey hit Houston on August 26 and lingered for the next four days, dumping so much rain on the city that streets were flooded and MD Anderson was forced to close. Nancy's Mobile doctors regarded the situation as sufficiently dire that she began chemotherapy immediately. We made it to Houston—finally—after a month of treatment that had done no good, though it left her so weak I was not even sure we could make the trip. I was terrified at what might await us.

The terror abated as soon as we met Dr. Kiran Naqvi, who would serve as Nancy's lead oncologist. Dr. Naqvi was in her forties, we guessed, a petite and kind-hearted woman from Pakistan who was one of the stars at MD Anderson. After consultations with her hospital team, and another round of testing, she recommended a drug called Decitabine, which was less debilitating than the standard poisons in most chemo. The goal, she said, would be remission, then a dangerous and delicate stem cell transplant, which could provide a cure. But if remission proved to be impossible—and she thought this was likely—the secondary goal was "stable disease," a high quality of life that would, she hoped, be measured in years.

Nancy and I embraced this plan; what else could we do, and our goal together was to celebrate every second of life, for as long as that life might last. We found that we enjoyed our "Houston Days," as we came to call them. On the eight-hour trips back and forth from Mobile, a dismal journey except for the beauty of the Atchafalaya Basin, we would listen to the news, or E Street Radio, and stop as needed for ice cream at McDonald's. Nancy's choice was an M&M McFlurry; mine was a soft vanilla cone, dipped in chocolate. There was nothing wrong with fast food, we decided.

Members of the family drifted in for visits—her daughter-in-law, sister, and son; her nephew, and two stepdaughters. Sometimes we would binge-watch "Grace and Frankie," and sometimes with Chris, the son she loved with all of her heart, we would sit quietly together watching golf. Sometimes I would leave so they could watch it alone. Once in Mobile, when she was feeling stronger, she and Tracy, the youngest stepdaughter, set off together on a shopping spree. I was their driver, but I never went with them into the stores. That was Tracy's domain. She was, by profession, a personal shopper and Nancy liked to tell the clerks in J Jill or White House Black Market that she had brought her fashion consultant with her. By Tracy's account, they laughed uproariously as they rapidly tried on clothes—laser focused before Nancy grew tired—searching for a wardrobe that might fit her. She had lost thirty pounds. "My all leukemia diet," she said.

Carolyn, her best friend since their days at Irwin Avenue, came in to oversee a redecoration of the house—a modest improvement in the feng shui, which I knew would go better without my involvement. So the weeks went by, and winter morphed happily into the spring. Dr. Naqvi changed the treatment once, from Decitabine to a trial drug known as Avulumab, and Nancy sent emails about these changes to friends and other members of the family. But mostly what she wrote about was life and the things that make it sweeter.

The other night I was walking our dog, Cooper, and was relieved to smell the honeysuckle blooming on the tangle of bushes along the side of the road. There is something about that delicious fragrance that is comforting and reminds me of my childhood. Learning to bite off the end of the blossom and suck the juice was a skill I passed on to my son and to our grandchildren. I assume all of you have similar memories that bring up those kinds of experiences. It's always the little things . . .

And on another occasion: *Have a great day tomorrow! Stay safe, wear your seatbelts, hug a friend or an enemy or both, and wave to the children in a school bus.*

By the spring, Nancy knew it was time to retire and on April 19, after she made it official, the leaders in the College of Education held a reception in her honor. Nancy was feeling strong and she gave a little talk. She said she was lucky—forty-eight years of doing what she loved—but now it was time for younger teachers to take up the baton. They also gave her the Excellence in Teaching Award presented annually by the college, and more than a hundred of her colleagues rose to applaud. Her smile was radiant. But later as we were driving home she reflected on the irony of receiving this award in a year when she had done no teaching at all.

"Well," I told her, "when it comes to the larger lessons in life, I think there are people who would beg to differ."

May was another good month, a happy time on the River. The pelicans and ospreys put on their show, skillful fishers that they were, and a family of mallards took up residence near the marsh. "I could get used to this," she said. But in June on our return to Houston, the bottom fell out. Inexplicably, the Avelumab had ceased to work. Nancy's blast count, the measurement of the fat and useless cells in her blood, which carried no oxygen and simply took up space, abruptly spiked to eighty percent. Dr. Naqvi prescribed a Hail Mary round of harsh chemo, and if it worked, a clinical trial on a new drug.

"How much time do I have?" Nancy asked, for the first time. "You can tell me."

"If these things don't work," replied the doctor, as gently as she could say it, "probably not a lot of time."

As we left the office I could see Nancy was stunned. I was too, but that seemed utterly beside the point. We walked to our car somewhere in the bowels of the eight-story parking deck, which was the only place of privacy we had before the chemo started in the afternoon. We sat together in the front seat and wept. We had not done this before. Not once. But now the grief came in a flood. I do not remember much of what was said, but I do remember she sobbed near the end, "Who is going to take care of you?" This was, I thought, always the default position of her heart, this unerring love for other people that was stronger in Nancy than anybody I had ever known. I remembered, improbably, a night in Charlotte when we had gone to a talk by Mother Theresa. We were surprised at how disappointed we were. This Catholic saint from the streets of Calcutta seemed to be such a bitter old lady. Nancy was not. After fifteen minutes she gathered herself and the two of us walked back inside for the Hail Mary poison.

Nancy suffered more in the next several weeks than at any other point in the illness: chills and fever, a weakness I did not expect her to survive. Somehow she did. By mid-July, as the chemo slowly drained from her system, they told us we could go home to the River. In two weeks, once it was gone, we would return to Houston for the trial drug.

Nancy was happy on the way home, and all the more

so when we turned into the driveway just after midnight. It was July 17, her 70th birthday, and a greeting in letters three feet high stretched across the front lawn. It was a gift from Chris and Jarin and Lincoln: HAPPY BIRTHDAY LOLLI.

Lolli was the name she and Lincoln had chosen.

The next morning, as we sat together on the porch, she said it was the best birthday of her life. Bur four days later she was so weak that even with my help, she could not walk from the bathroom back to the couch. An ambulance rushed her to Providence Hospital and she was admitted to intensive care. After a few more days in which I did not go home, her Mobile oncologist came in to see her.

"You should not go back to Houston," he said. "If you do, you will not make it back to Mobile. It's a matter of weeks. Maybe days."

As we absorbed the news together, Nancy was calm. She said it was time for Hospice. I called the family and two or three of her closest friends and told them they should come right away. From Durham and Portland and Nashville and Charlotte, from Boston, New York and Georgia, most of them were there by the afternoon.

We were lost in our thoughts, all of us, as we gathered in the waiting room at Providence. Chris was thinking of the quiet moments, the quality time, he and his mom had spent together, and thinking as well about how she had shielded us from the pain. She seemed so happy, so optimistic, even though she must have known what could happen. Jarin said later she remembered happy times— Nancy trick or treating with Lincoln on Halloween, then going to a party for parents in the neighborhood, dressed as a nun and drinking wine, dancing with everybody in the room. She knew Chris was right. Nancy was a protector of the people she loved, but she was also a person who refused to let leukemia rob her of joy. This was another of the lessons she taught in this rich and final year of her life.

On that same afternoon Rachel, her stepdaughter, wrestled with feelings of deep apprehension—almost a terror—as she approached the door to Nancy's hospital room. In one of their most recent conversations they had been chatting happily about Rachel's engagement to her partner Susan Shea. Now everything was rushing toward an end, and Rachel was nervous about what she would find.

"Rachel! Tell me about the wedding!" This was the greeting when she entered the room, and Rachel knew she should not have been surprised. This was Nancy. But the marvel was that she remained so utterly herself, so completely focused on the people around her, even as her body was giving way to leukemia. Later, she said with a contagious laugh, "This is one of the best times of my life. Everybody I love is here and I don't have to *do* anything."

Tracy would remember her own emotion in the warmth of welcome that greeted her as well. She and Nancy had talked or texted almost every day since long before the coming of the cancer. Now, in the fading light of this hospital room, she knew some might wonder about the depth of happiness on the eve of Hospice. Was it a façade? Tracy was sure that it was not.

She presented Nancy with a gift from Gemma—a ten year old's watercolor painting of a heart surrounded by the colors of a rainbow. She said Gemma was worried it was not good enough.

"Let's FaceTime her," Nancy announced.

To Gemma she said: "It's just *beautiful*, Sweetie. Thank you so, *so* much!"

Gemma was relieved.

Improbable as it seemed—even to me, the person who may have known her the best—this was the way it went for these last three days. That evening, after the ambulance ride back home to the River, Nancy rallied and for nearly two hours all of us gathered in the living room, laughing, telling stories, singing songs. Finally, as she sat in her wheelchair holding Chris's hand, she said she was tired and ready for bed.

"This is great," she added, by way of benediction. "Everybody should do this."

For the next two days her body grew weaker, but on the afternoon of July 27 she was hungry. "Carolyn makes the best scrambled eggs," she said, smiling toward her best friend. Happy for this unexpected assignment, Carolyn scrambled one egg and added some cheese. Nancy ate it all, and repeated the verdict: "The best egg *ever*."

In the late afternoon, she took a few minutes to text her grandchildren. To Ethan, who had wondered with the frankness of a twelve-year-old about how he would find her after she passed, she said he should look for a beautiful sunset. "I'll be there," she said. To Abby, the oldest, she offered gentle instructions: "Never forget how much I love you."

With Tracy, the youngest stepdaughter, about whose tender heart she worried, she invoked their mutual love of the absurd: "You have to be happy. Or I will haunt you."

As the final hours passed, I could still barely fathom the courage and generosity of spirit—the resolute good humor—that only seemed to be growing stronger. Nor could I fathom the cruelty of what she was having to face. I tried to keep the darker thoughts at bay.

That night we lay together in the bed and she looked over at me with the whisper of a smile, "I'm so happy," she said. I told her I loved her and I was too. Thirty minutes later she was gone. All of us were there with her. Little Cooper, the King Charles spaniel, lay on the pillow next to hers.

I knew in that moment, and the ones just before, that we had done what we set out to do. We had lived every minute that she had left as fully as they could possibly be lived.

But I also knew in this excruciating instant that I had no idea what happened next. I had given little thought— really almost none—to the shape of life without Nancy in it.

The Legacy

There were duties that had to be performed, of course. I remember sitting down at my computer and typing out an email to her family and friends and a note to her larger community on Facebook. She had written regularly to a long list of people—messages of optimism and hope that lifted the spirits of those who were worried. As I began to write about her death, I did my best to mimic her courage.

In a moment, to me of unfathomable sadness, Nancy Gaillard died last night after a yearlong encounter with leukemia. A lot of people describe such passings as the end of a fight. With Nancy it was more like a journey, a year full of joy and purpose and meaning. Against her spirit, leukemia did not stand a chance. Nancy was an educator—first a kindergarten teacher, then an elementary school principal, and finally an assistant professor of education at the University of South Alabama. She earned her doctorate at the age of 67. The University has established The Nancy Gaillard Love of Teaching Scholarship in her honor. But as determined and tenacious as she was, whether it was running a marathon or pursuing her career, these qualities of character came in second to Nancy's well of generosity and kindness. Today we went to the Dew Drop, a Mobile restaurant that is one of our favorites, and the young man who cleans the tables and knew of her illness because they were friends asked me how she was doing. When I told him, he said, "Oh man, that hurts my heart." Nancy read every chapter, every word, of my upcoming book, A Hard Rain, *and it is dedicated to her with love and gratitude. I am under instructions to take delight in its release, and I will try. In her final two days of life she was surrounded by family—her son, Chris, stepdaughters, Rachel and Tracy, daughter-in-law Jarin, and sister Harriett—and a few of her oldest and closest friends. She gave all of us, collectively and individually, our specific marching orders for happiness in her absence. We will try to heed her counsel but it may take a while. I join with other FB friends who have offered words of gratitude for her life. I am a lucky man.*

I posted the message and called the Hampton Inn in Houston where we planned to stay during her next round of treatment. This had been our motel of choice, and Nancy, of course, had befriended the desk clerks. She always liked people who did their jobs well, and was careful to let them know it. I recognized the voice of the woman who answered the phone (Nancy would have known her name, but I did not) and told her I needed to cancel the reservation.

"Do you want to reschedule?" she asked.

"No," I said, "Nancy died last night."

There was silence followed by a muffled sob.

"I can't believe it," the clerk said finally. "She was

always so happy and kind."

The conversation that followed lasted ten minutes, as other members of the motel staff came to the phone to offer condolences and snippets of memory about their interactions with Nancy. She was always so cheerful, they kept saying, even on our last visit when leukemia and chemo were taking their toll and she needed a walker to make it to her room.

"God bless you, Mr. Gaillard," one of them said. "You will be in our prayers."

That was the way it went in the weeks leading up to her memorial service, and the scattering of her ashes off the banks of Fowl River. Tommy, the man who cut our grass when Nancy was too weak for the riding mower (her favorite toy,) came by to let me know that he was feeling an inconsolable loss. Tommy and Nancy were friends. They always talked when he came to work, often about the details of his life, and Nancy loved to tell other friends about the time he was chopping at a tangle of vines, and came upon a snake. It was a water moccasin, but Tommy decided not to kill it. "I just didn't have the heart," he said. Nancy decided he was her kind of man.

"You know," said Tommy, with a catch in his voice. "Miss Nancy was like a sister to me."

I never knew why this tall and always grizzled man of middle age felt the need to say "Miss Nancy." I assumed it was simply a matter of deference, something propriety seemed to require as a ballast for affection that clearly went deep. "Tommy," I said, "Your friendship was very important to Nancy."

At the memorial service on August 22, I braced for the eulogy by our friend Steve Dill, a retired United

Methodist minister, ninety-one years old and ramrod straight, with a voice that reminded Nancy of God. We had first heard him preach on a New Year's Day at an African American church, not long after our return to Mobile. It was the anniversary of the Emancipation Proclamation and Steve had been asked by a group of black preachers to deliver the white apology for slavery.

"What in the world am I going to say?" he had asked a few days before.

"I have no idea," I replied. "But Nancy and I will be there to hear it."

On that New Year's morning Steve chose as his text the words from a venerated Negro hymn, "Were You There When They Crucified My Lord?" Obviously, he explained, none of us in the church that day were there at the crucifixion, but the words of the hymn compelled us to say: "Sometimes it causes me to tremble." He began to recount the racial history of America—the brutalities of slavery, the missed opportunities of Reconstruction, the ongoing cruelties of Jim Crow, and finally, in our current time, the racist realities that demeaned our system of criminal justice. After each topic, he paused to affirm: "Sometimes it causes me to tremble."

It was mesmerizing, and when it was over Nancy gave me an assignment. "You have to collect his sermons," she said, "and get them published in a book."

So I did.

This was the history Steve brought to the eulogy. As he gazed out across the people in the church, where the sunlight filtered through the stained glass windows, his voice as always was reassuring and strong.

Nancy's death was so devastating because her life-force is so resilient and her spirit so jubilant; it made her death more difficult to comprehend; the world assumed a certain strangeness; the very streets looked different. But even more peculiar, Nancy still seemed to meet us along the way. It was as if she ceased to meet us in particular places in order to meet us everywhere.

This eloquent man, so full of empathy and insight, also spoke about her career: "To Nancy education was a sacred trust."

I would like to say that I found relief in these testimonials, the powerful affirmations of Nancy's legacy and the all lives she had touched. It was true, of course, that I was grateful in the midst of grief—and less ambiguously I was proud, as if I had been married to a rock star. But the pain was simply too intense, and it came in waves— griefquakes, my daughter, Rachel, called them—that did not abate as the months went by.

I began to read C.S. Lewis' memoir of loss, *A Grief Observed*, about the death of his wife, Joy Davidman. Joy had been a brilliant poet who was first his friend then the love of his life. This sounded familiar, but so did the reality he now had to face. Before Davidman's death from metastatic carcinoma, Lewis said he never understood pain; now he found that he could not escape it.

I understood exactly what he meant. In 2019, after the first Christmas came and went without Nancy, I found myself in a very dark place. Issues of social injustice, which had always been a preoccupation (the by-product of being a Southerner), now took on a magnified intensity that was simply not healthy for my psyche or heart. I became obsessed with stories about family separation—

the cries of children on our Southern border, torn from their asylum-seeking parents in a cold-eyed national policy of deterrence. I knew Nancy had grieved about it too. These were children, after all. Suddenly, I felt a perfect storm of despair, as if my pain were intermingled with her compassion, and all of it with the anguish of families who had sought sanctuary in the land of the free.

About the same time, for reasons that made no particular sense, I picked up a copy of *The Diary of Anne Frank*, the journal of a Jewish teenager hiding in an attic, while the Nazis outside were trying to kill her. Nevertheless, she was able to write: "I still believe that people are really good at heart." Two weeks after that journal entry, on August 4, 1944, the dreaded knock on the door finally came, and the Franks were arrested and taken to Auschwitz. Anne's mother and sister did not survive, and Anne, herself fell victim to typhus. In the United States, a theology student named William Hamilton was trying at the age of nineteen to process the magnitude of the horror. "I wrote out my two choices," he remembered. "God is not behind such radical evil, therefore he cannot be what we have traditionally meant by God," or "God is behind everything, including the death camps—and therefore he is a killer."

By the 1960s, Hamilton had emerged as a leading theologian in the Death of God movement. In the first year after Nancy's death, I found myself drawn to this theology of gloom. I don't mean that I compared my personal loss to the Holocaust; of course I did not. But somehow the perpetual cascade of pain left me pondering the suffering in history—and the worldwide anguish in our own time—in a way I never had before.

It was depression in the form of political rage, and I tried to keep the depths of it to myself. Not that there were not reasons for rage. I knew then, and continue to believe, that we were living in a sorrowful time. But it occurred to me, oddly, in the middle of it all that Nancy would be worried about me if she knew. I was struggling without her steadiness and wisdom—not to mention the pursuit of fun—that had been the staples in our relationship.

It so happened that in these months, I was working on an article for *Alabama Heritage*, a historical quarterly published by the University of Alabama. It was a piece I called "The Rabbi and Dr. King"—an account of the warm and philosophical friendship between Martin Luther King and the Jewish theologian, Abraham Heschel. In the 1960s, they were allies in the civil rights and antiwar movements, and I thought as I started to read Heschel's writings that Nancy would have loved him. He often raged with the fury of a prophet against the suffering he saw in many places. "Our thoughts about Vietnam are sores," he wrote, "destroying our trust, ruining our most cherished commitments with burdens of shame. We are pierced to the core with pain . . ." But he was also a man who paused every day to give thanks for the mystery and beauty of life, who came at the world with a twinkle in his eye. God, he thought, was not an omnipotent puppeteer, pulling the strings of human history, but a personal presence in a world full of hurt, who needed the help of human beings to heal it.

As I finished this article, I began to reflect on the shape of my career—an inclination that Nancy had supported to write about problems in American life through the stories of people who tried to make them better. And so I decided to write about Nancy. I had gotten an email from Lauren Templeton, a graduate student at South Alabama who had been picked as the first recipient of the Nancy Gaillard Love of Teaching Scholarship. She told me that she had been a student of Nancy's at a difficult time. She was a single mother going to school full time and working three jobs while trying to care for a sick child.

"Dr. Gaillard," she wrote, "came into my life at one of the lowest points…On that first night of class, she picked me out like I was a sore thumb—noticing how worn down I was. She continued to check on me and ask about my daughter even after I was no longer her student. She was kind, full of sunshine, and I met her at a time I needed her most. She told me not to stop in life until I was happy."

Almost as if somebody had planned it, other notes and emails trickled in as well. I knew I was lucky to have the support of good friends. Many of them were Nancy's friends too, and they were scattered from Alabama to Tennessee and New York, from the Carolinas and Georgia, to Florida and the coast of California. Lynn Smith-Loving was one of those, and she wrote me more than once with thoughts about Nancy.

"It was easy to underestimate her," Lynn said. "She was so positive, so happy, so loving. She embraced her husband, her friends, her students and most everyone around her with enthusiasm. It was easy to think that she wasn't discerning. That she didn't see the very real weaknesses in all these people. It took a while to understand how complex her embrace was. To understand that she really did understand our faults, but loved us anyway."

In the course of this correspondence, I began to see the story I wanted to tell. It was a love story, of course. How could it not be? Love was the animating force of Nancy's career. If Steve Dill was right, and I think he was, that education for her was sacred, it was a mission pursued in every life she touched. But she also saw the larger implications, all the inequality, injustice and hurt that could shackle and wound the life of any child. She knew the great transformations many of us hoped for were beyond the reach of any one teacher, any single person in any line of work. But she could try. She could embody the opposite of all that was wrong with every bit of love and strength she could muster.

Perhaps the greatest test of that understanding came in the final year of her life. She knew from the start that her form of leukemia might well be fatal. She simply refused to let it change her. I am in awe—everybody who knew her remains in awe—that she was able to succeed even through her closing minutes of life.

"I'm so happy."

The words, even now, continue to astonish.

And so we come to the redemption of the writer—a husband more prone to darker emotion. I wanted these reflections to be more than cathartic, the story of a teacher as well as a wife. I knew that's how she would want me to tell it. But I make no apology for the healing it brings, slow and uncertain as that may be.

If the road after Nancy is twisting and hard and still full of hazard, I have come to see as I write these pages the direction I know she would want me to go. One thing I learned in the course of thirty years. She was generally right about these things.

Part II. *Last Letters*

During her illness, Nancy wrote regular notes and letters—emails mostly, and occasional texts—to family and friends. She wanted to reassure the people who loved her. She did not share much about the physical discomforts that went with her treatments; nor did she talk about them often in private. Only in the rarest of moments did her defiant optimism disappear.

There were intervals when she was weakened by chemo and didn't feel up to writing but did not want loved ones left in the dark. She asked me to pinch-hit. On those occasions, I tried to take my cue from her—and her powerful inclination toward hope. As I say in the last of these emails, "against her spirit, leukemia did not stand a chance."

This was the way she approached the journey. It does not take a lot of imagination to see how such generosity and good cheer might have meshed with her career as a teacher. And in terms of the larger lessons of life, many of us thought, Nancy's time with leukemia may have been her finest hour.

As I read these letters again, I am struck once more by the great good fortune of my life. I am also stunned by the magnitude of the loss.

In Nancy's words:

August 30, 2017

Dear Friends and Family,

Just to catch you up on my progress with my adventures with my new diagnosis of AML (acute myeloid leukemia). This is a brand new thing for me—being "sick" and having to stay confined for a month or so. I have had fatigue and difficulty breathing for about a month and after many, many tests, this is what it is. I feel sorry for my wonderful nurses and doctors and Frye who have to remind me that I can't be the energizer bunny. But I am doing well, don't panic—I'm not going anywhere; it just changes my lifestyle. So rather than sending a bunch of individual texts and emails, I am going to keep all of you posted on my progress. This way you will know that I am still kicking ass and what delightful adventures I am having.

So here goes:

Day 1

Enter Providence Hospital, room 1241, no flowers, fruits, raw veggies, or anything that might bring spores or pesticides, etc. Bummer!

Lots of tests to get ready for chemo.

Good meds for nausea and infection given through I-V.

Started chemo—regime of 7 days—24 hours a day—called an induction—then 3 days of additional meds to help kill bone marrow cells—then just watching and waiting for signs that my body is reproducing good cells.

I was supposed to go to Houston at MD Anderson to do all of this but clearly with Hurricane Harvey, that is impossible. So I will go there for phase 2 of treatment later on.

I feel good. Crappy stuff begins in a few days. Bring on the long red wig! Frye has been and is being fabulous. I have so many of you who are nearby who are willing to do anything and I know those of you who are away are supporting me with good vibes! Those are so important. We are not going into crisis mode. This is just a problem to be solved. Houston is a crisis!!!

So take care of yourselves. Thank goodness for football!

Roll Tide Roll!
I love you all!
Nancy

August 31

Friends and family,

No excitement here. Just learning to live with my chemo cart and how to maneuver it as I walk, shower, and try to stay active.

Food is not bad and I can order outside food if I want to. Best news is that I can keep a cooler here with adult beverages (don't tell).

Hematologist says my platelets are dropping which means the chemo is doing its job. That is good.

I talked to folks in MD Anderson in Houston and they hope to be up and running again by Tuesday. I won't go there until I finish this month's round of treatment. I spoke at length to the nice lady who called to check on me and she and her family survived the flooding. She seemed to appreciate the fact that we asked about them.

I want to send very special thanks to my friends and colleagues at USA in our College of Education and Professional Studies (CEPS) for covering my classes and taking care of our students. We are a very fortunate group of educators to have each other.

Nurses and doctors here are magnificent. I was moved today to a different room that has a little room off to the side for more space. Like our college, they work together as a team to provide care and concern for each other and their patients.

I hope all of you are well and ready for a good weekend. Frye and I appreciate, more than you know, all of the kind thoughts, prayers and well wishes.

Best always,
Nancy

September 1

Finally a break from daytime TV with the start of football. I think I will become a fan of every team. I may even start keeping stats. (Never thought I would use that word again. Statistics was not my favorite course.)

Hope everyone is in weekend mode. I continue to get chemo and have named my chemo cart Ida—for the medicine that goes through it—Idarubicin. Ida and I walk daily around and around the nurses' station in the hospital pod where I am temporarily living. We figured out today that 35 times around the station is a mile. I figure I will work up to that point by adding a round each day.

I do not wish to purchase this suite I am in. But it isn't too bad for a short-term lease. You might want to look elsewhere if you are interested in Mobile real estate. Just saying . . .

No big news. I still have hair although the plan is to become a bit more hairless on Wednesday. I shall not send a picture. Much too scary for the faint of heart.

I continue to get excellent care. And I can never thank all of you enough for the kind thoughts, prayers, and good vibes. I feel them every minute of every day. I'll take the weekend off and continue writing on Monday. You guys need a break. Meanwhile . . .

Go Heels! Go Jags! RTR! Go Panthers! And just to show you how generous i am feeling, WDE! If you have no idea what I'm talking about, just ask any Alabama resident or look it up. Nothing like it anywhere!

Love you all!
Nancy

September 4

Happy End of Labor Day Friends and Family! Hope each of you have actually observed the "no-labor" rule—a very odd designation . . .

I thought about this day's name all day as a continuous group of very talented and hard-working staff members came in to do their jobs without complaint, without a scowl, and with the same good spirit that I have seen every day here. One person stands out. She came in to clean the room and I said I was sorry she had to work today. She looked at me and said she did not mind and she works seven days a week—weekends at the hospital and cleans a local elementary school the other five days. Not easy work or fun work—but oh so important work. Be sure to thank the person who does this kind of work wherever you are.

Have a great day tomorrow! Stay safe, wear your seatbelts, hug a friend or an enemy or both, and wave to the children in a school bus.

Love you guys,
Nancy

September 6

Woo hoo! Last few hours of this first round. Thank you for hanging in here with me.

I think my body has finally said, I'm tired and leave me alone. But just starting this adventure. So much more to come.

Will make an appointment tomorrow at MD Anderson for early October for second opinion about what to do next. We've heard so many wonderful things from so many of you about the excellent work they do. The folks here are so good and caring and I may be able to continue some treatment here.

Prayers and good thoughts for all of you who are being affected by Hurricane Irma and other coming storms. We can always help others if we are spared.

Have a good night. Love you all,

Nancy

September 7

Good evening Friends and Family

Hope you have each survived your day and are staying safe from pending weather, fires and other tragedies that stretch across our country. Now is the time for us to work together—regardless of our own politics, prejudices, and other foolish things that divide us.

Things I have learned to bring for a lengthy hospital stay:

> Hair dryer
> WD40 for squeaky wheels
> A beloved who reminds you NOT to sit on your PICC line
> NOT Jim Cantore
> REAL TOILET PAPER

Other than that, I am happy and relieved to know I am in good hands.

TAKE CARE OF YOURSELVES TONIGHT and through the weekend wherever you are.

Peace,
Nancy

September 10

Dear Family and Friends,

I'm pinch-hitting this evening, writing in deference to the patient's end of the day fatigue. It was another pretty good day, all in all. The room can feel like Grand Central Station with all the nurses and doctors doing their jobs, managing the possible chemo side effects before they have a chance to gain momentum. These folks continue to be conscientious and kind.

Biggest news of the day: The Day 14 bone marrow biopsy to determine how close we are to remission. While these procedures are not something Nancy would do recreationally, she insists—amazingly, convincingly—that they are no big deal. We hope to know some results within a few days. We will, of course, keep you posted. Meanwhile, as Nancy reminds me, prayers for those in Irma's wake . . .

Love to all of you,
Frye

September 11

Greetings Friends and Family of Nancy,

Sorry but it's just me again. The patient has asked me to pinch-hit due to her fatigue, which hits pretty hard this time of the day. That being said, Day 13 was a good one—the third in a row after a rotten day last Friday. The doctors are pleased with how it's going and Nancy continues to receive EXCELLENT care at Providence Hospital in Mobile. Her sister Harriett, whose home in Thomasville, GA is somewhere in the wrathful path of Irma, is still here and bringing an extra professional eye to the whole process. I, myself am upholding the first principle of the Hippocratic oath: Do No Harm.

As we may have said, we will be headed for MD Anderson on October 2, and sometime midweek this week, there will be another bone marrow biopsy to see how close we are to remission. We will keep you posted. Meanwhile, Nancy continues to inspire us. Thanks to all of you for your thoughts and prayers. Keep 'em coming.

Love,
Frye

September 14

Dear Friends and Family of Nancy,

It takes more than leukemia and chemo to keep this girl from having a good day. Round 2 has begun and while we know that it will be tough, Nancy and I had as fine a morning and afternoon of hang-time as two people can have. Sister Harriett has returned to Georgia to attend to her own life, and we appreciate her caring and medical knowledge. Nancy's son Chris arrives tomorrow for a brief visit, and after that Nurse Ratched (that would be me) has proclaimed a moratorium on guests until this round of chemo is over and we can assess the side effects and results.

Please keep Nancy in your thoughts and prayers and feel free to email or text if the spirit moves you. She misses you and looks forward to actual sightings in the not distant future. Thanks for your love and concern,

Frye

September 18

Greetings everyone,

Nancy has begun the fifth and last day of the second round of chemo, and I'm happy to report she's hanging tough. She's exhausted from the rigors, but still managed several laps around the nurses' station today in the company of her rolling IV chemo dispensary. Because of the miracles of another drug, Zofran, Nancy has experienced only a moderate amount of nausea, which has helped to make the ordeal bearable. Her fever has spiked a time or two as expected, but it's a symptom controlled so far with Tylenol, and though she has begun to lose a bit of hair I'm happy to report she looks way cool in a baseball cap. As for her spirits, she is just amazing. I've always been a little in awe of my resolute and beautiful wife, but never more so than in the last month.

We don't know exactly what happens next, or what medical strategies might lie ahead, but we will continue to keep you informed. Nancy appreciates you more than you know. We loved having Harriett and Chris here last week, and there are so many people she would love to see. Thanks for understanding that for a while longer she just can't do it.

In closing, Nancy asks me to ask you to remember others in need with your prayers, particularly our neighbors in the Caribbean. It's unbelievable that some of them are about to be hit with their second category 5 hurricane in a matter of days. So many natural and manmade disasters. We just have to keep on keeping on.

With gratitude,
Frye

September 20

Dear Friends and Family of Dr. Nancy,

We may slow down the frequency of these reports so as not to wear out your in-boxes, especially if, as we hope, things settle into a routine. But I wanted to let you know that today was a good day at Providence Hospital. Nancy has begun to regain a little strength with the second round of chemo behind her. She sat up in her chair all morning and made several laps around the nurses' station, which was a significant improvement from the day before when getting to the bathroom was an ordeal. She is determined to do her part to keep up her strength, and it's safe to say that the doctors and nurses are pleased as they can be with her resolve. We are in a waiting game now. There will be another biopsy next week, which will help determine where we go from here, and as of now we are expecting to travel to Houston for an appointment at MD Anderson on October 2.

Meanwhile, her care at Providence continues to be excellent. During our conversations today, it occurred to Nancy and me that we should mention, among the other caregivers, the housekeeping crew that keeps her room clean. Orlando and Sade and the others do their jobs with great conscientious and care, and with a kind of cheerful spirit that can't help but make a patient feel better. It may well be that nobody grows up thinking, "gosh, I hope one day to be able to mop floors and scrub toilets at Providence Hospital." But the truth is, those kinds of jobs matter and no place more so than at a hospital. Those of us who are lucky in life can so easily overlook the people who do these important things well, but this kind of illness gives you time to reflect and to appreciate the good people around you. Which includes all of you who are reading this note.

Thanks as always for your support,

Frye

September 25

Hey everybody,

A good report at the close of the day on Monday. Nancy was pretty uncomfortable on Sunday but has felt better today, even though she is still zapped after the two rounds of chemo. The doctors are conferring tonight about next steps. I hope we'll be headed for MD Anderson this weekend, assuming she is strong enough to travel, and there we'll enter the next phase of treatment, It's a journey and we're on it together. Thanks for being with us,

Frye

September 26

Dear friends of Dr. Nancy,

The Mobile doctors have conferred and the plan is this: Nancy and I head for Houston on Saturday; she rests on Sunday, and enters MD Anderson on Monday, 9:00 sharp. We'll postpone the biopsy originally scheduled for today until she gets to Houston since they'll do one there. Sometime fairly soon we should have an idea what form of AML (her type of leukemia) we are dealing with and what kind of additional treatment is needed. Two rounds of chemo intended to stop the cancer in its tracks temporarily are now complete and have certainly exacted a physical toll on Nancy's energy. But she rested comfortably today after walking her laps around the nurses' station. Though I admit to a bit of bias, I grow prouder of her determination every day, and we both remain grateful to all of you. (Some things bear repeating.)

Thanks again,

Frye

September 28

Dear Friends,

Plans are confirmed. Barring something totally un-expected, Nancy comes home tomorrow (Friday) from Providence Hospital and we set out for MD Anderson on Saturday morning. We were talking this afternoon almost wistfully about her time at Providence, such has been the quality of her care. Out of appreciation, Nan-cy decided we should send a cake to the nursing station with our gratitude inscribed in icing, and our friend Wendy at the University of South Alabama took care of the details. One of the nurses, who has probably spent more time with Nancy than anyone else, came in and gently kissed her on the top of the head. "I have fallen in love with you," she said. (This was not a creepy gesture, you understand, not inappropriately familiar, but rather an act of pure sweetness. And of course, it is not hard to fall in love with Nancy.) We are both a little anxious about the trip. Nancy's white blood cell count seems to be close enough to normal to afford her some immunity from random microbes, but her energy level is SO low. And of course, we don't know precisely what's ahead. What we DO know is that everybody we've met who has had any contact with MD Anderson—and the number of people is surprisingly large—offer nothing but the most superlative praise. So we are moving forward with hope.

Again, our love and gratitude,
Frye

October 2

Hello friends,

A final report before the weekend. Nancy began a new regimen today with a powerful and highly effective chemotherapy called Decitibine, which has been the highest standard of care for complex leukemia in people over the age of 60. She is taking it as part of a clinical trial comparing the effectiveness of a new drug not yet on the market with Decitibine. By random selection, Nancy is part of the control group taking the proven drug. Her doctor, Dr. Kiran Naqvi, who is wonderful, is confident that either drug holds great promise in Nancy's case. This treatment will continue for five days on an out-patient basis, so Nancy is able to come "home" to our suite at the Hampton Inn. We will confer again next Thursday with Dr. Naqvi. Nancy is feeling good. Have a great weekend.

Thanks to all,

Frye

October 13

Dear Friends,

Nancy has finished a five-day treatment of Decitabine at MD Anderson. The drug has an excellent record of putting Nancy's complex form of leukemia into remission and her brilliant doctor believes it may take three or four treatments, maybe more. We will be returning to Houston for those with the next one scheduled for Nov. 6. Multiple blood tests each week will occur between treatments. Nancy also met with the stem cell team at MD Anderson and if the team follows her doctor's recommendation, she will receive a stem cell transplant as soon as she achieves remission, probably sometime next year. The transplant is a rigorous process, but MD Anderson does more than 800 every year with a very good rate of success. It will be a long road, but we have the best team in the world to go along with Nancy's deep determination and resolve, and both of us feel good about the increasing clarity of our path.

Thanks for traveling with us,
Frye

October 27

Dear friends,

This Friday morning did not start out well. We had a doctor's appointment already scheduled for blood work and Nancy barely had the strength to get there. We had to use a wheelchair to get her inside the building. As we suspected, the blood work revealed that her hemoglobin was low—a common symptom with leukemia, and one we had not seen for several weeks—so it was no surprise. But the effects were as severe as any we've had. Fortunately, two units of blood did their thing and for the rest of the day Nancy has felt much better. She most often uses a walker. She can get around without it, but it's handy for balance. Her spirits are just fine, but today was a reminder (like we needed it) that it is going to be a long haul.

And then there's this: When I went to pick up dinner tonight at the Pelican Reef, our neighborhood seafood dive, the whole wait staff came over to ask about Nancy. They usually do. At the CVS Pharmacy earlier in the week—one of the busiest chain pharmacies in Mobile—two of the pharmacy staff people came up to the window while I was picking up a prescription. "You tell your wife," they said, "that we love her to pieces." At the Dew Drop, a hamburger place where we eat a lot, our friend Addie, who has long been a favorite waitress, always asks about Nancy. Earlier this week, so did the busboy, a young African American man who doesn't talk much, but who really likes Nancy. All of this means a lot to her. And me too, of course. It reminds me of what I have learned from Nancy about the importance of treating people well. So thanks everybody for your support. Nancy feels it everyday.

Happy weekend,

Frye

November 17

I'm back! Thanks to Frye for pinch-hitting the past two months when the chemo had me pretty exhausted.

It has been a good day! Spent a few minutes in an actual store and sat in the Publix cafe while my wonderful sister shopped for us. She is such a gift and we continue to laugh and enjoy old and new times together. With advice from Walt (her son) and Chris, we are binge-watching the Netflix series, Stranger Things. Oh boy! It's really good!

The latest good news from MD Anderson is that they have found two perfect (10/10) stem cell donors for me. We are very hopeful! If I can just get into remission and have good heart and lung reports... There are other possibilities if needed. We feel confident and positive about the road ahead. We have much to be thankful for. Celebrate early and often this football weekend! Be safe!

Love,
Nancy

November 30

Happy Thursday to everyone!

Hard to believe it's the last day of November and still such beautiful weather here in Mobile. Our leaves are just showing color while I know that some of you are already into winter. Wherever you are we hope you are well.

I'm doing just fine and gaining more and more strength each day. Folks here at the Southern Cancer Center continue to monitor my blood and make certain that I am getting what I need. They treat all patients with care and maintain a positive attitude. I'm beginning to get to know the nurses and some of the patients. It is true that this cancer thing forms a community. The same is true at MD Anderson where we go on Sunday for Cycle 3 treatment. My son Chris will meet us there and come with me to appointments on Monday. I look forward to having him there.

Here's to December, football, family, friends, and hope for our country. Let's all contribute to better understanding and choices in whatever way we can. I think it's up to us now!

Much love to everyone and always gratitude for your support.

Nancy

December 6

Dear Friends,

We are in Houston for cycle 3 of Decitabine and doctor appointments. It was wonderful to have my son Chris here to see the place where his mom comes once a month and to meet Dr. Naqvi and her team, who are taking such good care of me. Chris has been so attentive throughout this journey along with all of you. As always, Frye is my caretaker and chief "listener" when we go to these appointments. He is so good at remembering what is said and makes certain I do what I am supposed to be doing. My brain isn't the best during these times (a good excuse). I am very grateful.

Today was day 3 of the treatment with no ill effects. I am gaining strength each day and walking without the aid of a walker. This is a huge improvement although I am a bit disappointed I don't need the "Cadillac walker" with a seat and brakes. We see the stem cell doctor Friday and should have some blood-work results. No bone marrow biopsy this time (you can imagine how upset I am) but will save that pleasure for January's visit. We head back to Mobile Saturday.

Frye and I wish you the best and will keep you informed during the holidays. This is such a difficult time of year for many, in addition to the joy it brings as we celebrate and ponder our blessings, of which there are so many. Don't lose sight of those blessings and do what you can to help those in need, not just this month but every day of the year.

Peace and love to you and your family,
Nancy

January 15

Happy Tuesday to Everyone!

On an icy day, I'm happy to report that Frye and I are now in an apartment in Houston for the next month while I continue to receive treatment. I have been in the hospital for a week and have finished the first cycle with no ill effects. I can't begin to describe how wonderful the nurses and doctors and staff were to us. Many of the nurses appeared to be about 12 years old, which indicates how old we are. But their skills and demeanor are just what a patient and family needs.

I will continue to get blood work done regularly to monitor my progress, and will get another dose of the trial drug on the 22nd. Dr. Naqvi and her team watch me closely and remain hopeful that this treatment will be effective. Our fingers are crossed.

We were thrilled to have Jarin, our daughter-in-law, while Frye had to travel for a few days. She and I wandered around the hospital and found some incredibly lovely spaces for resting and hanging out. The observation deck on the 26th floor gives a panoramic view of Houston and the surrounding areas. Another area called The Park provides a beautiful spot with plants, soft chairs, a coffee shop, gift shop, and (for the holidays) a display of gingerbread houses made by various groups in Houston. These are examples of how MD Anderson strives to make everyone feel hopeful. Superb leadership creating a positive community in any organization.

Please take care of yourselves and stay warm and safe in the cold weather. We love you!

Nancy

January 21

Dear All

It's Monday and the weather in Houston was just spectacular today! Beautiful blue sky, 70 degrees and folks walking around in shorts. My kind of winter! Hoping wherever you are it is equally as nice. I do love Southern winters.

A multitude of thanks to my wonderful sister Harriett for coming to help me nest in our apartment while Frye had to return to Mobile for business and to receive the Arty Award for the outstanding literary artist in 2017! A much-deserved award. Believe me, at this point in my life I do need an entire tribe of helpers and I am very grateful for the support from everyone. My energy level is good but I do tire easily and need moral support when I realize that both age and AML can wear one out.

Frye and I saw Dr. Naqvi today and she is very pleased with my ability to handle the new treatment protocol. Thus far, no ill effects (knock on wood), and my appetite is better than it should be. I have even been known to sip a glass of wine. So . . . I bring everyone greetings from Houston and MD Anderson, one of the most incredible institutions I have ever seen. There are so many folks much worse off than I am but everyone here seems to remain in good spirits.

Peace, love, hope, and belief in all things kind and good,

Nancy

February 20

We arrived home late last night to beautiful weather and the warmth of winter in the deep South. We love it! And we love the fact that the doctors here and in Houston continue to treat us with respect and dignity and with such positive attitudes. I am very fortunate! There are no positive indications that the current treatment is doing it's job but it often takes many cycles before blast counts are getting lower on a regular basis. I am not discouraged. I am blessed with all of you as my friends and with a wonderful husband who is by my side every step of the way. I am so glad he continues to do his own work, which is so very important to the literary world. His new book on the 60's (A Hard Rain) is absolutely amazing.

Again, take time to appreciate the little things in life. They are so important to you and to everyone else. The events of the past week should remind us that we have a responsibility to each other and to teach our children, speak to our politicians, and get involved in our communities about what is necessary to live peacefully together.

Blessings to you!
Nancy

March 21

Good Wednesday Evening to everyone!

The calendar has declared it Spring so it shall be! I realize some of you are NOT as fortunate as those of us in LA (Lower Alabama) so I won't rub it in, but this is that time of year when we sneeze constantly with pollen from pine trees and other budding vegetation. It's the time when Lowe's and the local growers put out their bedding plants and that particular shade of bright green almost hurts your eyes. We will, inevitably, have one more cold snap but who cares? The seasons continue.

Frye and I are in Houston for two days (we head back home tomorrow) for my 14th day dose of Avelumab, the trial drug. Then we have a couple weeks off before we return for the next round of treatment. The labs show I am still in good shape with blood work—no news yet on blasts (the bad cells)—but I will have another bone marrow aspiration in April and that may give us an idea of how this trial is working. I feel great and have energy and eat way too much. But that's okay. My bikini days are long gone (thank goodness) and I enjoy every day.

Thank you for your continued support and kind words and thoughts. Please share them with others as well. It becomes contagious and then it really helps everyone.

Love to all!
Nancy

April 6

The other night I was walking our dog, Cooper, and was relieved to smell the honeysuckle blooming on the tangle of bushes along the side of the road. There is something about that delicious fragrance that is comforting and reminds me of my childhood. Learning to bite off the end of the blossom and suck the juice was a skill I passed on to my son and to our grandchildren. I assume all of you have similar memories that bring up those kinds of experiences. It's always the little things . . .

Frye and I head back to Houston on Tuesday for a week of treatment. I will have a bone marrow aspiration Wednesday, hopefully giving us some idea of how this trial drug is working. We know it may take a lot more time so we are prepared. Life here on the river makes up for any anxiety or impatience. I have no pain or discomfort and receiving blood every 2—3 weeks keeps up my energy level. It's all good. Enjoy night walks this week. Take care of each other. Try something new.

Cheers.

Nancy

May 1

It's May Day friends! Hopefully you are beginning to see warm weather and signs of hope that winter is over. Take it all in!

Musings that brought a smile while on my walk tonight with our faithful dog, Cooper . . .

Lighting bugs (fireflies) in the sweet-smelling magnolia trees

Our feral cat "Mama Kitty" walking with us and talking the entire time

Our neighbor's Christmas tree still lit and reminding me that it SHOULD be a year-round feeling and message of hope and love

The last remnants of a spectacular sunset

Our thanks to our daughter-in-law, Jarin, and grandson, Lincoln, who visited in Houston, and to my sister who came to Mobile to hang out and take me shopping. My sincere thanks go to out to my colleagues at USA's College of Education and Professional Studies for allowing me to be a part of a fabulous learning community for the past 14 years. Today is my official retirement date and I can't believe how fortunate I am to have worked for 48 years doing what I love to do. I am a very lucky lady.

We return to Houston next week for another round of this trial. Our neighbors take care of our critters and the house and we are so very grateful for all they do for us. My doctors here in Mobile and in Houston are pleased that my leukemia is "stable" and that my general health is good. They emphasize that immunotherapy results do not always have the goal of remission, but do have the goal of maintaining good quality of life. I'll take that any day!

Take care of yourselves and those around you. Keep a smile on your face.

Be kind,
Nancy

May 25

Home from two weeks in Houston to happily blooming flowers after plenty of rain here on the river. And
more to come this weekend if predictions are correct. A
wonderful friend brought gardenias by the house today
and their fragrance as well as the magnolia blossoms at
night remind me how lucky I am to live in this part of
the world. I even found a lone zinnia blooming in the
garden—a reminder that last year's flowers continue to
revive themselves. There is always hope.

Reports from Houston are good. My lab results are
stable and my doctor is pleased with my progress. I will
have another bone marrow aspiration the first week of
June. This should help determine if we will continue the
trial I am currently on or if we should look for a new
one. Frye and I are pleased that there are many options
for treatment and we continue to trust our team of phy-
sicians and nurses who are optimistic and supportive.

Happy almost summer to all of you. Take good care
of yourselves and don't forget to smile, laugh, and be
kind.

Nancy

July 7

Musings from Houston:

It's hot here—no beautiful river to make it feel better

Fire alarms in our hotel at 2 a.m. bring people close together (there was no fire) and interesting choices of clothing for nightwear (we all laughed)

People drive as if there are no rules

Weekends at MD Anderson are much less hectic than during the week

There are a lot of very nice people who work at this hotel who take seriously the whole idea of kindness for all people

Updates for medical news:

I've received some pretty high-powered chemo, which has left me fatigued and what little hair I had rapidly falling out again. Had another bone marrow aspiration yesterday, which should help determine the next course of action. Thanks to so many family members who have come to visit during these months and stay with me while Frye has had some work to do requiring travel. We may be able to come home in a week or two. I miss our beautiful spot and our fur babies. But thanks to our neighbors, I know they are in good hands.

So hope everyone is enjoying summer and vacations and family and friends. Continue to be kind to everyone, even those with whom you disagree, and help each other. Frye and I love you and appreciate everything you do for us. Carry on!

(On Nancy's birthday, she exchanged emails with her stepdaughter, Rachel. The heading on Rachel's note to Nancy was, "To My Wicked Stepmother," a standing joke, initiated by Nancy, with both her stepdaughters.)

Dear Nancy, who is the very model of step-parenthood and who has suffered under a ridiculous misnomer,

There is nothing I could think to give you for your magnificent 70th birthday that would come close to what I really want, which is just some way to tell you how much I love you and how grateful I am that you are one of my parents. No physical gift can do that, so I decided to take the usual family route and to write it down.

Almost since I can remember, you've been there, encouraging me to find my own path and celebrating my achievements and dreams with me. Every time in my life that I have shared a story or a decision with you, from whether to audition for a play in middle school or what to major in in college or where to move for graduate school or how to raise my children or how to plan my own midlife second wedding, you've been there with support and enthusiasm and interest and wise counsel. I trust you so much and think I should have told you before now how closely I carry your advice and your love, and how much I think about both and always have. Sometimes in reaching out to you and sometimes in just knowing I could, I have always found you a safe harbor.

I can just as easily think of you singing "Rock and Roll Girls" in the car with the wind blowing and your head tipped back as I can see you calmly and firmly helping a child regain his footing after a meltdown or talking to a parent who needs both guidance and a firm limit. If I were really doing this right, I would have dug through the disaster that is Abby's room after her frenzy of packing for camp and unearthed her giant sunflower head, and I'd be wearing it while I type. You are my favorite blend of fun and wisdom and silliness and compassion and determination.

You taught me how to be a stepparent. Everything I've ever done right in that role is because of your love and your example. I bring you into my parenting all the time, too, and I could not have asked for a better grandparent for Abby and Ethan. They love you so much, and Corbin and Hayden do, too.

I know on big birthdays we tend to reflect on things, and I didn't want this one to pass without my sharing the reflections I carry around with me every day about you. You're one of my favorite things about the world, and I love you.

Happy birthday.

Love,

Rachel

Dear Rachel,

Oh my. There is no better gift than this. I will print it and keep it with me always. You are such a fine woman. Your parents did well and I'm just so happy and fortunate to have had a chance to be a part of that. Please make every moment count. I know you will. I love you! Never forget it!

Nancy

July 24

(This was Nancy's last email, written to her friend and colleague, P.J. Danneker, whom she met at the University of South Alabama. P.J., not knowing Nancy's condition had worsened, had written earlier in the day about new friends she wanted Nancy to meet.)

Dear PJ,

What a find!!! But I think, my love, that it's over for me. I've done enough crazy stuff. My body is done. Just can't talk right now. Love you dearly. I'm in Mobile at Providence Hospital and will be until I go home with Hospice. I love you man!!

July 28

Dear Family and friends,

In a moment, to me of unfathomable sadness, Nancy Gaillard died last night after a yearlong encounter with leukemia. A lot of people describe such passings as the end of a fight. With Nancy it was more like a journey, a year full of joy and purpose and meaning. Against her spirit, leukemia did not stand a chance . . .

Love,
Frye

Part III. *In Memoriam*

At Nancy's memorial service on August 22, 2018,
her three children—son, Chris; stepdaughters Rachel
and Tracy—delivered their reflections on her life, speak-
ing for the family. As you will see, they spoke from the
heart. How they got through it, I was not sure. There
were tears involved.

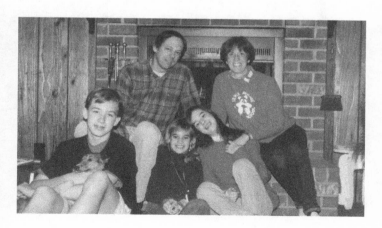

Rachel Gaillard Smook

I had the opportunity this summer to participate in a workshop given by a singer-songwriter named Connor Garvey, who writes what he calls "acoustic funky-folk-rock for the good-hearted." He ended it by playing a song he'd written called "Tattered Shirt," and it brought Nancy immediately to mind. The song begins:

I am my mother's daughter, and most can tell
They say it is a likeness of the eyes
Less of the color, more how we see
The beauty in what's cast aside
So bring me a vase of dandelions and Queen Anne's lace
Bring me a heart that's torn and tired
And I will love you, I will love you, I will love you.

Nancy understood the beauty in what's cast aside, and she loved it all. I have a fondness for lilies and lilacs, but Nancy's favorite flowers were daisies. There is a patch of them at the edge of my yard that has been blooming ferociously this summer. I'm fairly sure I would have overlooked them, except that Nancy's love of them taught me not to, so instead I purposefully stop and notice them now. I pay attention to their bright petals and sunny centers, and I photographed my daughter in their midst to capture an image in which everything in the frame is beautiful.

A child in the daisies: what could be a better snapshot of the things that Nancy loved? Her reverence for children was simply unparalleled. In every picture I have of her with her grandchildren, she is beaming, and they've spent their childhoods rich in the absolute certainty of her devotion. They are all so different from one another in personality and in passion, but Nancy celebrated each of them as individual miracles. She deeply knew and truly understood them all, and she delighted in them. And while adoring one's grandchildren is something we might expect of a loving grandparent, it was bigger than that for Nancy. She celebrated every child, including those whom life and circumstance had cast aside. She believed inherently in their value and worth, and she helped them believe as well. She guided parents and teachers and students in upholding and honoring the sacredness of all the children with whom she came in contact, and of those she never met. When I think right now about how impossible it feels to me to comprehend a world without Nancy in it, I am comforted by the thought that thousands of children and countless teachers carry her with them and keep her influence alive and thriving.

I was a child when I met Nancy. She called herself my wicked stepmother, which is of course preposterous. No child has ever been luckier in a stepparent than my sister and I were. Nancy loved us as her own. On her last morning, I bent down to offer her a sip of water, which she declined, but she took my hand and looked right into my eyes and said, "It has been the joy of my life to have two daughters." I will hear those precious words in my head again and again for the rest of my life, and I am so profoundly grateful. Because of Nancy's absolute acceptance and love, I never experienced being part of a stepfamily as anything but a benefit. She told me when she married my dad that she would never try to be my mom, but she loved us so much that she became one of our parents despite herself. She taught me that whatever changing shape a family takes, it is a place of comfort, support, advocacy, and most of all unflinching love. I will tell you with certainty and gratitude that anything I have ever done right as a stepparent myself is because of her example. Corbin and Hayden, it is part of my life's best work to be as devoted to you as Nancy was to me. And Abby and Ethan, as our own family has changed shape, I want you to remember that I learned from the best, and that I brought Gramma Nancy's lessons with me into my choice about who I trust to love you as we all move forward.

Nancy and I were talking the day before she died and I said, "You're still teaching me stuff," to which she responded, "I always will." I'll ask you to stop and think about that for a minute, the notion that she is still teaching us, and that there's simply no end to what we can learn from her. Every time we bring her to mind, every time we consider what her actions would be as we choose our own, every time we act on behalf of children whom the world has cast aside, every time we take a step toward shifting this world in a kinder direction, we will honor her, and she will teach us for as long as we are willing to learn.

For my part, I will also stop to pay attention to daisies—and lilies, and lilacs, and dandelions, and Queen Anne's lace. I'll look for the best in children no matter their state or circumstance. I'll love deeply and say so often.

My heart right now is torn and tired, but I am so grateful to be one of the people Nancy loved. I hope that for the rest of my life I will be forever recognizable as her daughter, because of a likeness of the eyes: less of the color, more how we see.

Chris Frederick

At home, the board members of the company I work for often joke that I like to get the bad news out of the way first. After Mom passed, I was trying to help in whatever way I could. Trying to get the bills in order was one of those ways. Going through folders and various loose papers, I came across a recent Houston hotel bill that was eight pages long and the only charges were the cost of the room and the taxes. Also included just below the hotel bill was the weekly trending of results from her laboratory tests.

These lab results were like her report card. Only it wasn't math or English or history or PE. It was the report card of life at that moment. I came to the conclusion that Mom knew what was going to happen to her—that was the bad news—but she shielded us from that, knowing the pain it would cause. She did not want to spread that pain. Thinking now about her life, I can imagine no more honorable to way to be remembered than as a "Protector of Others." Throughout her life that's what she was, and these "Others" included the thousands of children who walked the halls in her schools; the teachers she mentored both as a principal and later in life during her second career at the University of South Alabama. And throughout her sickness she has protected her family and friends from the reality of the situation through her positive outlook, incredible attitude, smile and gratitude for her time here.

During her illness, I texted her every day when I exercised. This was our daily check in. I have really missed those texts these last three weeks. Now on this day of her

Memorial Service, I want to thank all of you for being here. It is truly impressive and very comforting to our family. So thank you to those who have travelled and spent money so you can be present to remember her: to friends and family, and the brave young people who may be experiencing this for the first time, and have even less understanding of how to come to grips with it than the adults. And a special thank you to Frye who has put his life on hold to be my Mom's caregiver throughout her illness.

While my Mom was a teacher in the classroom, she was also a teacher as a parent. I remember one Sunday I refused to get dressed for church. She said that is fine; you can get in the car and go to church wearing your pajamas. I stubbornly rode to church in my pajamas and she called my bluff in the parking lot. Needless to say I changed my clothes in that parking lot and went to church fully dressed.

Her work ethic was unbelievable. She was no nine-to-fiver. She would work twelve-hour days, attend my sporting events, come home and lesson-plan for the following day. She was a tireless worker who was dedicated to making others better. I remember during her first retirement speech after thirty-three years in the Charlotte-Mecklenburg school system, she apologized for missing out on much of my life. I had no idea what she meant or why she made this apology. We went to the beach every summer. She never missed a game of mine. I was able to tell her shortly before she passed that I had no idea what she talking about when she apologized on that day. She squeezed my hand and asked if was sure. I am grateful to have had the chance to erase her concern.

I will always remember my trips to Houston and Mobile to be with her during her illness. It was probably the best quality time we ever had. We watched entire golf tournaments. Not really knowing much about golf, she would ask me about all of the game's crazy rules. She pulled hard for one particular golfer to win a major tournament. It was fun to share that. Surprisingly, she was also a big fan of boxing, and we would stay up late watching entire boxing matches.

There was a moment at Mom's house on Fowl River that I will cherish forever, and knew I would the moment it happened. I was fishing off the pier. And I use the word fishing very loosely since I have to use a glove to take a fish off of the hook to throw it back. Mom was sitting on the pier in her chair and said that for her whole adult life, her friends had told her she needed to slow down and quit working so hard. She told me she finally knew what they meant. The sun was shining on her as she stared up at the sky in her Alabama baseball cap. She took this huge deep breath and let out this high-pitched sigh of relief. I had seen firsthand my Mom "at peace."

Carolyn, my mom's best friend for over forty-five years, recently sent me a two-word text with those same words, "at peace." It confirmed what I had witnessed and it was wonderful. My point is, please do not feel sorry for us. We are at peace because Mom was at peace.

I realize how extremely grateful I am for the last few days that I and others got to have with her. Not everyone has that opportunity, and I feel for those who have lost a loved one without it. There are a few moments over her final days that stick with me. She told me, perhaps as a grandparent to my son, the importance of teaching independence. I am relieved that she is now independent of her cancer that she fought so bravely. I was able to tell her that she was an incredible mother. I played sports year round and felt so supported when she attended my games. All of them, despite her long work schedule. It was great to remind her of this as a father who understands how challenging it can be.

Alabama is definitely football country. My mom texted me RTR—Roll Tide, Roll—before every Alabama game. I will miss those texts. Where I live in North Carolina, it is basketball country, and the loyalty to UNC basketball is the closest equivalent to the loyalty to football in Alabama. There are two UNC alumni here. Mom's best friend, Carolyn, is here. As is Mom's sister Harriett. Years ago, my Mom and Harriett reconnected. Harriett thank you for that. My Mom absolutely loved your beach trips to Destin to laugh and tell stories and just be with her sister.

In keeping with the theme of sports, I want to say that my all-time favorite speech came from Jim Valvano, the legendary coach at UNC's rival, North Carolina State, who was battling cancer. He spoke about the disease and never losing sight of what life is all about. It's a message that is as important today as the day Jim Valvano first delivered it.

"I'm going to speak longer than anyone else has spoken tonight," Valvano said, accepting the first ESPN-created Arthur Ashe Courage Award. "Time is very precious to me. I don't know how much I have left and I have some things I would like to say." What he said was essentially a blueprint for living a full life, and for cutting through all the bullshit the world might hand you:

"To me, there are three things we all should do every day of our life. Number one is laugh. You should laugh every day. Number two, think. You should spend some time in thought. Number three is you should have your emotions moved to tears . . . Think about it. If you laugh, you think, you cry, that's a full day. That's a heck of a day. You do that seven days a week, you're gonna have something special.

"Cancer can take away my physical abilities. It cannot touch my mind. It cannot touch my heart. And it cannot touch my soul. And those three things are going to carry on forever."

No wonder my Mom loved that speech.

Tracy Gaillard Pendergast

"Tell me, what is it you plan to do with your one wild and precious life?" These were the closing lines of a beautiful poem called "A Summer's Day," written by Mary Oliver. I read it in college and fell in love with it. Back then it spoke to me about the limitlessness of opportunity and the future, along with a reminder to go after the adventures, not wait for them to show up. It was perfect for a pithy, inspirational yearbook quote to boot. I've kept it in my mind for all the years since, but as of this summer, it reads much differently . . .

Losing Nancy has changed the way I see lots of things. Along with the overwhelming heartbreak, the omnipresent ache of missing her, there are the marching orders she gave us—to seek joy, find the fun in little things, to look out for each other, along with the profound obligation to honor her by sharing the kindness she offered so readily. She gave each of us so much from her wild and precious life, and we have a job to do to pay it forward.

Nancy was something special to everyone in this room, and many who can't be here. To my dad, she was his best friend, his cheerleader, his literary wingman and muse. With good reason, I think, they were so proud of one another. There is a passage in his recent book about the 1960's, *A Hard Rain*, that tells a story about Nancy's hero Mr. Rogers that I'd like to share. Mr. Rogers was someone who believed wholeheartedly in the value, the potential, the WORTH of every child, every human being, just like she did.

It begins here:

*Even a publication as urbane as Esquire magazine pub-
lished a profile of Rogers that was tinged with unmistakable
awe. Writer Tom Jurod recounted the time when Rogers went
to visit a boy in California, who was 14-years-old and severely
afflicted with cerebral palsy. The boy couldn't speak and com-
municated through a computer and sometimes with flailing
gestures of self-hate, hitting himself with his awkward fists,
telling his mother that he wanted to die. 'He was sure' wrote
Jurod, 'that God didn't like what was inside him any more than
he did.' Over the years, the boy had endured stares of disgust
nearly every time he left the safety of his home, and cruelty in
the form of verbal abuse, but there was one thing that gave him
comfort each day. He watched Mister Rogers' Neighborhood.*

*When Mister Rogers came to see him, however, the boy
was caught in a wave of self-doubt, feeling apparently that he
was unworthy. He began flailing and hitting himself again,
and his mother had to take him into another room to help him
calm down. And then, wrote Jurod, this is what happened:*

*. . . when the boy came back, Mister Rogers talked to him,
and then he made his request. He said, 'I would like you to do
something for me. Would you do something for me?' On his
computer, the boy answered yes, of course, he would do anything for Mister Rogers, so then Mister Rogers said, 'I would
like you to pray for me. Will you pray for me?' And now the
boy didn't know how to respond. He was thunderstruck.*

*Thunderstruck means that you can't talk, because some-
thing has happened that's as sudden and as miraculous and
maybe as scary as a bolt of lightning, and all you can do is listen to the rumble. The boy was thunderstruck because nobody
had ever asked him for something like that, ever. The boy had
always been prayed for. The boy had always been the object of
prayer, and now he was being asked to pray for Mister Rogers,*

*and although at first he didn't know if he could do it, he said
he would, he said he'd try, and ever since then he keeps Mister
Rogers in his prayers and doesn't talk about wanting to die
anymore, because he figures Mister Rogers is close to God, and
if Mister Rogers likes him, that must mean God likes him, too.*

Mr. Rogers didn't regard himself a hero for the way
he approached the child. He believed in earnest that
children, especially those who knew suffering, had a real
connection to God, and if they chose to share it with him,
then he was the lucky one. No wonder Nancy liked him
so much. They were the same. Nancy felt lucky to dedicate her life to teaching. Her students, from Kindergarten
to college, loved her, I think partly because they knew she
loved THEM, respected them, believed in them. Nancy
had a way of making anyone feel heard and feel special.
The leukemia robbed her of her wish to be an organ do-
nor, one of its many cruelties, but it gives me comfort
to think that everyone she taught, in the classroom and
beyond, is carrying a little piece of her heart with them.
If we're really lucky, they're asking themselves, What
Would Nancy Do?

When Nancy walked in to her office at the University of South Alabama, her favorite greeting was "GREAT
NEWS EVERYBODY, I'M HERE!" delivered with arms
outstretched and her famous beaming smile. She meant
it to be hilarious, and it was—the very idea that Nancy could be self-important or boastful in earnest was
preposterous. But I loved hearing her say it, not just because it meant you'd get to hear her laugh right after. I
loved it because she was right—it was GREAT NEWS
when Nancy appeared. It was like opening up the curtains
and letting the sun in—things just got a little lighter, a little

brighter. Since I was a little girl, she always made me feel like the hardest things weren't impossible anymore, because she had my back, and, somehow, she always understood. No wonder I told her all my secrets. She kept them all, listening with the selflessness and focus I really hope I learn one day.

Nancy's friendliness and warmth were her trademark. She's been described, more than once, as *unfailingly* kind, *relentlessly* optimistic, *indefatigable* in her goodness. When you lose someone, it is customary to speak of their best attributes. With Nancy, that means celebrating ALL of her, because she was THAT GOOD. Along with my profound grief, I feel profound gratitude for the friendship she gave me, the love she shared with my dad, and the family she made me a part of. I actually don't know how we're meant to function without her here; that is just too big a hole to fill. But I do know that in our own wild and precious lives, if we get a little lost without her, we have her legacy to guide us. The best way I know to honor her is to try and pick up where she left off, spreading the kindness and the light she shared without limit. With so many of us that love her, we don't have to go it alone.

Letters of Tribute

After Nancy's death and memorial service, notes and tributes came in a flood, some by email, some in the mailbox, others on Facebook and other social media. Nearly two years later, there is still a trickle. This is a sampling.

Mike Letcher—Emmy-winning producer-director, who adapted Frye's book, Journey to the Wilderness, *into a documentary film:*

"As I collect my thoughts about Nancy, the most obvious, of course, is the amazing serenity and perspective with which she approached the end of her life. I don't think one can do that who is not truly wise. Who does not see the world from very far *away*. Who does not see herself and her own life from very far *away*. By which I mean to see it as truly and fully as we can. In as much context and perspective as is humanly possible. And that takes a lifetime of complex contemplation and a desire to find meaning and to be meaningful.

"Nancy seemed to me someone who was an authentic listener, fully intent on connecting with you in the moment in conversation or shared experience. Fully present. There is a lot of graciousness and giving in that, and I think we always recognize and appreciate it when we are the recipients of it from others. And I think of it as consistent with her nature as a person who found much of her meaning in giving—as a teacher, as a friend, in all her relationships.

"I remember one instance that was particularly memorable and meaningful for me personally. During one of our visits to film 'Journey to the Wilderness,' I had a conversation with her in the back yard while Frye was inside tending to other things. I confided in her that I felt a connection to Frye, and to her, that transcended the professional rapport that one seeks to cultivate in the business of writing about or documenting a subject. I confessed that I thought it might be premature, presumptuous, self-serving or a kind of social climbing, but that it felt real. She recognized it as a vulnerable moment and assured me in the most genuine and convincing way that it was appropriate and truly reciprocated. It was a lovely, meaningful moment that I remember warmly and often.

"On that same trip, we took a ride in the Miata, a two-seater sports car I sometimes drove, which she thought sounded like fun. I appreciated her capacity for frivolity and joy around that little episode, especially when I let her drive. And it reminds me also of what I took to be a complete lack of pretense, a great sense of humor and a love for all things that are funny, fun and connect us all to one another in the most fundamental way.

"To the extent that one can measure the way in which a human life is lived, I think it has to be said that Nancy did it right."

Mary Letcher — wife of Mike, teacher, musician:

"I didn't know Nancy but in a fleeting sense, but it sort of didn't matter. She was pretty easy to know. What I mean to say is, for me, Nancy seemed to be someone you experienced. If I may, she was a *verb*, and a beautiful one. A lovely woman of quiet, reliable goodness that made you feel wonderfully whole. I know it may seem odd that I got all this from the few times I was with her, but I did."

Tom Lawrence—lawyer, friend of Nancy's and Frye's, writing on behalf of himself and his wife, former television journalist Carolyn Lawrence:

"In our relationship with Nancy, we knew less about her actual experience and impact as an educator than we did about the heart and soul of Nancy as a person.

"Our thoughts are concentrated on Nancy's unique human qualities, such as her omnipresent happiness and optimism, courage, and discipline. In terms of her career and ability as an educator, those qualities, among many others that she possessed, were cornerstones of who she was and therefore of what she brought to those she was teaching. Truly great educators couldn't exist without those qualities.

"We remember a weekend together at the River she loved—three families, old friends, with ties going back so many years—and how it serves as a microcosm with Nancy's beautiful self on display, always laughing, always generating ways to squeeze every drop of fun out of life for all of us, energetically making it happen but making it look effortless.

"We think of the unique combination of courage and discipline, and extraordinary passion to learn and to learn how better to teach, that led her to achieve her doctorate at a time in life when most ordinary humans were content to maintain the status quo.

"And any overview of our thoughts could not be summarized without all of these things coming together, along with her phenomenal courage, as she took that final journey, and did it, astonishingly, with a smile—which is beyond comprehension to most of us mere mortals."

Lynn Smith-Loving—friend of Nancy's and Frye's, professor of sociology at Duke University:

"Many people get less interesting as you understand them. Nancy was the opposite . . . I remember when my niece's husband had just died from liver cancer, and she and her children came down to Dauphin Island on the Alabama coast for a previously planned family trip to the beach. We had dinner with Frye and Nancy at their favorite haunt, the Pelican Reef. Somehow the conversation, which included a 10-year-old girl who had just lost her father, turned to dancing costumes and Halloween. Nancy suggested that peacock feathers would be just the thing to make a headdress. And guess who had access to peacock feathers from Bellingrath Gardens, where she had friends on the staff? Nancy.

"A couple of weeks after my niece and her daughter arrived back to their empty home in Tennessee, guess what came in the mail: Two very carefully packed peacock feathers. Can you imagine how hard it is to pack a peacock feather to make it through the mail to a little girl? My niece told me much later that she couldn't believe the kindness of a new acquaintance who remembered a promise to a little girl and followed through on it. My niece was astonished. Those of us who knew Nancy better weren't surprised at all."

Susan Santoli—Nancy's department chair in the College of Education and Professional Studies at South Alabama:

"We have a picture of Nancy hanging in our front office. It is a beautiful photograph capturing her in a pensive mood . . . Those of us who knew Nancy don't need a tangible reminder of her, but we want to share her with new faculty who come into our department. She would have been so thrilled at the young people we are hiring and would have been such a mentor and encourager.

"I have the same photo on my computer as my screen saver and it is blown up to life size, so I look at her face to face when I come in to my office, put my palm against hers, and I tear up every time. Her sweet, sweet spirit permeates our whole college and rarely does a week go without someone commenting on something Nancy did or said. Oh, to have Nancy's laugh bottled so that I could uncork it every day. I am so honored to have known her—her courage, her commitment to students, her true interest in all people—she was such a precious creation of God."

Laney Andrews—former graduate student at the University of South Alabama:

"Nancy was like a second mom to me during my grad assistant days and spent hours and hours encouraging me in my career. Some of my favorite memories were when she would visit me at school and compliment my teaching endeavors. She cared so much about the true meaning of education—the child! She always had a kind word, an infectious laugh, and a good piece of chocolate."

Peggy Delmas—teaching colleague South Alabama:

"I had the good fortune of having Nancy Gaillard as my next-door office neighbor for several years. She was funny, kind, and thoughtful. Sometimes Nancy would come to my office for a chat. After the 2016 U.S. Presidential election Nancy was a great comfort to me. Sitting in my office she would listen calmly to my anger, disbelief, and fear. She was a good listener at a time when I needed someone to hear me. Her humor, sense of peace, and perseverance bolstered me.

"Nancy was given to walking around the office barefoot. She also did things others might consider silly, like wearing a giant spider hat on Halloween all day at the office and then on an airline flight. I admired how free and confident she was.

"Sometimes Nancy walked laps around the interior of our building for exercise. As she warmed up, she would take off a layer of clothing and hang it on the door to our office suite as she walked by. If I entered that door and there was a sweater, scarf, or button-up shirt (or sometimes all) hanging on the doorknob, or piled on the floor I knew that Nancy was walking laps. I often wondered what the students thought of the bits of clothing that sometimes appeared outside our office.

"I was always impressed with how considerate Nancy was consistently. When leaving the office to go to lunch or run an errand she never failed to ask if I would like her to bring back some lunch or if she could do anything for me while she was out. She always asked, and it wasn't just a polite gesture. She really would have followed through.

"Nearly two years later, now that we are in the midst of a pandemic, I could use Nancy's calm, steady presence. It's not that she could necessarily do anything to counteract the awfulness of the world. But she made me feel better just by being in it."

Acknowledgements

This book is a work of non-fiction, part profile, part memoir. Some of the anecdotes and stories are based on my first-hand experience. For descriptions of events where I was not present, I have relied on the memories of family, colleagues and friends. Nothing is invented.

For the writer, this is sensitive terrain and the balance between too much emotion and too much restraint is delicate. In trying to find it, I have been guided by the goal of doing right by the subject. If the result is a portrait of almost unfathomable generosity and kindness, animating a life's work in education, then I have succeeded.

Thanks to the following people whose memories, love and support have made the effort possible:

Family and Kin: Chris Frederick, Jarin Frederick, Lincoln Frederick, Rachel Smook, Abby Smook, Ethan Smook, Susan Shea, Hayden Shea-Meadow, Tracy Pendergast, Gemma Pendergast, Mike Pendergast, Walt Bost, Andrea Bost Rogers, Harriett Loehne, Clay Smook, Norris Frederick, Julie Suk, Julie Whiting, Becky Toulmin, Ma'on Adams, Anne Adams, Rosemary Peduzzi.

Nancy's Work Family: Carolyn Bush, Steve Houser, Sherrie Faulk, Dryw Freed, Beth Leo, Debra Davis, Kristin Horner, Paige Vitulli, Andi Kent, Susan Santoli, Karyn Tunks, Abigail Baxter, Benterah Morton, Kelly Byrd, Peggy Delmas, Joel Lewis, Rob Gray, P.J. Danneker, David Johnson, Tony Waldrop

Mutual Friends: Tom Lawrence, Carolyn Lawrence, Ted Fillette, Ellen Holliday, Lynn Smith-Loving, Miller McPherson, Marti Rosner, Anne E. DeChant, Erin Shim, Cynthia Tappan, Steve Dill, Ruth Dill, Brenda Overcash, Allen Cowan, Vivian Lord, Mike Letcher, Mary Letcher, Robin Harvey, Julie Brickman, Laura Jamison, Steve Trout, Kent Rush, Becky McLaughlin, Claire Cage, Susan McCready, Randall Williams, Suzanne LaRosa, Wayne Lord, Rosa Lord, Barbara Filion, Kathryn Scheldt, John Dowdney, Roy Hoffman, Patti Callahan Henry, Gail Willis, Jay Westbrook, Melody Westbrook, Jerry Smith, Rachel Smith, Marilyn Craig, Justine Burbank, Ann Lertora.

The Doctors: Thanks finally to Dr. Kiran Naqvi and all the nurses and staff at MD Anderson in Houston, a place that sets the standard for cancer care, not only in their level of expertise, but in every warm and life-affirming detail that makes it a patient-friendly place: the paintings and photographs hung on the walls, the waiting room aquariums brimming with brightly colored fish, the kindness of everyone who works there. Thanks also to Dr. Brian Heller and the nurses and staff at the Southern Cancer Institute in Mobile, and the medical staff at Providence Hospital. As Nancy's last letters make clear, from the professionals who clean the hospital rooms, to the nurses, to the doctors, she received the best possible care. She was grateful. So am I.

About the Author

Frye Gaillard is Writer in Residence at the University of South Alabama. He is author of the award-winning titles, *A Hard Rain: America in the 1960s*; *The Dream Long Deferred: The Landmark Struggle for Desegregation in Charlotte, North Carolina*; and *Watermelon Wine: The Spirit of Country Music*.

CPSIA information can be obtained
at www.ICGtesting.com
Printed in the USA
BVHW030912221120
593766BV00003B/11